THE FIGHT FOR
PUBLIC HEALTH

THE FIGHT FOR PUBLIC HEALTH

Principles and Practice of Media Advocacy

Simon Chapman
Department of Community Medicine, Westmead Hospital,
Westmead, New South Wales, Australia

Deborah Lupton
Faculty of Humanities and Social Sciences, University of
Western Sydney, Nepean, New South Wales, Australia

BMJ
Publishing
Group

First published in 1994
Reprinted 1996
by the BMJ Publishing Group, BMA House, Tavistock Square,
London WC1H 9JR

British Library Cataloguing in Publication Data

A catalogue record for this book is available
from the British Library

ISBN 0-7279-0049-9

Typeset in Great Britain by
Apek Typesetters Ltd, Avon House, Blackfriars Road, Nailsea

Printed and bound in Great Britain by
Biddles Ltd, Guildford and King's Lynn

Contents

Preface

I began my public health career as a health educator in 1974, working for one of the many Australian Government drug abuse prevention programmes that proliferated in those days. After a few years of devising educational packages about perspectives on drug use, "values clarification" and even "how to say no to drugs", conducting teacher training workshops and provoking furrow browed civic fathers to think more about their alcohol intake, it became very evident that these sort of approaches were largely piecemeal, often pointless, and ultimately pathetic. We were a handful of earnest idealists just spitting into the wind of the real determinants of drunk driving, diazepam dependency, and teenage cigarette use. Whatever aggregated little gains we might have made in changing community knowledge and attitudes, these were swamped day after day by major structural determinants of drug and alcohol abuse such as price, licensing policy, and especially the promotional activities of the tobacco and alcohol industries. Together with a few equally disillusioned colleagues, I helped form a pressure group in 1978 called MOP UP (Movement Opposed to the Promotion of Unhealthy Products). We met in a cheap Sydney Lebanese restaurant and sat about bemoaning the futility and myopia of a fixation on what people would later describe as "downstream" or "host directed" approaches to public health problems.

Our major achievement was to cause the Australian comic actor Paul Hogan (later to star in the *Crocodile Dundee* films) to be barred from advertising Winfield cigarettes because of his enormous popularity with children.[1] This victory took 18 months, climaxing in four of us sitting in a tension filled room before the chairman of the national Advertising Standards Council, along with the grey faced chief executives of the Rothmans tobacco company and their hired expert witnesses. When the verdict was announced, The *Australian* newspaper's front page headline read "MOP UP's slingshot cuts down the advertising ogre", an allusion which captured one of the most enduring themes in public health advocacy: the David and Goliath struggles of small, ill equipped community groups representing issues of social justice against giant and wealthy behemoths in industry or government. The stones loaded into MOP UP's slingshot during the 18 months included the strategic use of research (we conducted a survey of cigarette brand preference among 12–14 year old smokers); humour (we held our first public meeting in a forensic sciences lecture theatre attached to the city morgue); and the creative use of expert advice (we had a professor of psycholinguistics provide a statement about the ordinary meaning of the critical term "major appeal" in one of the Advertising Standards Council's clauses after Rothmans argued that "*major appeal* [my emphasis] to children" could not also mean "major appeal to adults", Hogan being popular with all age groups).

Quite easily our most important weapon, however, was the way we framed ourselves as Davids against the Goliath of the tobacco industry. This allowed us to appropriate a whole tradition of journalistic interest in the fortunes of the underdog: to become fodder to the perennial question: "Can a little group on the side of the angels beat a big group that sups with the devil?" Our non-institutional status also allowed us to remove the restraints of the guarded, conservative public commentary that, as daytime Government employees, we would have been obliged to observe had we spoken about the issues in our "official" workday capacities. Our small group rapidly became identified by sections of the Australian media as a reliable source of forthright comment on related public health matters.

This process was for me the beginning of what has developed into a career in public health advocacy which, over the years, has caused me to wear enough hats to open a millinery shop. I have been active in public health advocacy, particularly in the tobacco control and gun control fields, via involvement with MOP UP (long since disbanded), the international consumer movement through the Australian Consumers' Association and IOCU (the International Organisation of Consumers Unions) through the British Medical Association,[2] the Australian Public Health

Association, the Australian Coalition for Gun Control, and especially through my work as a university researcher and teacher. In this last role, I have been extremely fortunate to work since 1987 with Stephen Leeder, Professor of Public Health and Community Medicine at the University of Sydney. Steve has continually encouraged me to see my advocacy work as a legitimate and important part of contemporary public health practice. Rather than marginalise it as some sort of informal, extracurricular part of academic work, Steve has instead encouraged me to promote its importance alongside more established public health areas of study such as epidemiology, disease control, health education, and health economics.

The idea of this book grew out of a series of short courses on public health advocacy that I coordinated and taught in 1991–2 in four states of Australia, joined by Rebecca Peters, Don Nutbeam, Phil Wilbur, Alan Blum, Steve Woodward, and John Cornwall, former Minister of Health in South Australia, following a grant shepherded through the bureaucracy of the Commonwealth Department of Health and Community Services by the perspicacious Liz Furler. Following these courses, I began teaching in public health advocacy in the Master of Public Health degree course at the University of Sydney. It quickly became obvious to me that here was a classic instance of a missing public health text: there was very little that could serve as a text that would guide students through the core issues of advocacy principles and practice. However, towards the end of our writing this book, a work was published on media advocacy and public health by Larry Wallack and his colleagues at the University of California at Berkeley.[3] Based almost exclusively on American case studies, their book is a very useful and recommended companion book in this field.

Deborah Lupton, my co-author, is one of the leading analysts of media issues in public health in Australia. She has collaborated with me on several papers and research projects examining the social aspects of medical and public health issues,[4-8] and is the author of recently published books on AIDS reporting[9] and the sociology of health and illness.[10]

Finally, there are too many people to thank and acknowledge as important influences on my thinking about advocacy. A long list would commence with names such as Stan Glantz, Peter

Vogel, Arthur Chesterfield-Evans, David Simpson, Phil Wilbur, and Mike Pertschuk. Two people, though, deserve special mention. My friend Rebecca Peters, a former Sydney radio news producer, lawyer, and fellow advocate for gun law reform, has taught me a great deal about what it is like to work in a news organisation. As a news producer and an advocate for a public health issue, she has had the benefit of both gatekeeping what gets through to the public as news, and what it is like to try to have a public health issue given the coverage it needs. If you have a friend like Rebecca, your learning curve in advocacy will rise very steeply. Steve Woodward, former head of Action on Smoking and Health (ASH) Australia and now with ASH in London, is without hesitation, the most tenacious, perceptive, and imaginative public health advocate I know. I have worked closely with Steve and there are very few tricks and moves in the book of advocacy that I have not seen Steve demonstrate with a master's touch. He could name his price with the tobacco industry, but, fortunately for us, the currency he values is in very short supply with them.

Simon Chapman
January 1994

References

1 Chapman S. A David and Goliath story: tobacco advertising in Australia. *BMJ* 1980; **281**: 1187–90.
2 British Medical Association. *Smoking out the barons. The campaign against the tobacco industry*. Chichester: John Wiley & Sons, 1986.
3 Wallack L, Dorfman L, Jernigan D, Themba M. *Media advocacy and public health. Power for prevention*. Newbury Park: Sage, 1993.
4 Lupton D, Chapman S. Death of a heart surgeon: some thoughts about press accounts of the murder of Victor Chang. *BMJ* 1991; **303**: 1583–6.
5 Lupton D, Chapman S, Donovan B, Mulhall B. Attitudes to and use of condoms amongst multi-partnered heterosexuals in Sydney, Australia. *Venereology* 1992; **5**: 41–5
6 Lupton D, Chapman S, Wong WL. Back to complacency: AIDS in the Australian press, March–September 1990. *Health Educ. Res. Theory Practice* 1993; **8**: 17.
7 Chapman S, Lupton D. Freaks, moral tales and medical marvels: health and medical stories in a week of Australian television. *Media Information Australia* 1994; **72**: 94–103.
8 Lupton D, McCarthy S, Chapman S. Panic bodies: discourse on HIV risk

among people who have sought testing. *Sociology of Health and Illness* (in press).

9 Lupton D. *Moral threats and dangerous desires: AIDS in the news media.* London: Taylor and Francis, 1994.

10 Lupton D. *Medicine as culture: illness, disease and the body in Western societies.* London: Sage, 1994.

Acknowledgements

We are grateful to the following: the Public Health Research and Development Committee of the National Health and Medical Research Council, Australia and the National Heart Foundation for grants in 1993 to study the news on public health and heart disease respectively; The Advocacy Institute, Washington DC for making available material for sections of Part II (see page 130); Judith Watt and the Health Education Authority, London, for making available copies of the British health news reportage described in Chapter 3; the publishers of *Media Information Australia*, for permission to publish an edited version of "Freaks, moral tales and medical marvels: health and medical stories in a week of Australian television" in Chapter 3; the publishers of the *Australian Journal of Public Health* for permission to publish an edited version of "Children's lives or garden aesthetics?" (co-authored with Victor Carey and Daniel Gaffney) in Chapter 4; the BMJ Publishing Group for permission to publish an edited version of *Tobacco Control* 1992; **1**: 50–6; the Australian Medical Association for figure 2; Annie Stiven and Louise Helby for coding the news study described in Chapter 3; Ron Davis; and Peter Vogel for figure 7.

I: Theory and principles

1: What is public health advocacy?

SIMON CHAPMAN

In December 1992, the Australian parliament passed legislation that banned the last remaining forms of tobacco advertising in Australia.[1] The rot for the local tobacco industry set in first in 1976, when the Australian Government followed the examples of countries such as Britain and banned direct advertising of cigarettes on radio and television. This meant that print, outdoor, cinema, and point of sale tobacco advertising remained, along with the growing trend to promote cigarettes "indirectly" via the sponsorship of high profile sporting and cultural events.

Arguing that it was impossible to be half-pregnant, public health advocates sustained their attacks on these remaining forms of advertising. They argued that if the Government agreed that radio and television advertising of tobacco should be banned because it promoted smoking, then they were bound to agree that these other forms of advertising also promoted smoking, and so logically should also be banned. Between 1976 and 1992, these remaining forms of tobacco advertising began to tumble, domino style, under a sustained programme of lobbying and advocacy. With radio and television being out of bounds to the tobacco advertising dollar, the commercial print and outdoor advertising media and sections of the sporting and cultural fraternities began receiving literally tens of millions of dollars annually in advertising and sponsorship revenue from the politically influential tobacco industry. These groups soon developed both a financial dependence on the industry for operating in the ways to which they had become accustomed, and an

3

understandable sense of gratitude towards their benefactor. The threat of forced divorce at the instigation of public health advocates raised great concern that they would be unable to find such bountiful support. The result was that the tobacco industry's opposition to a proposed ban on print media advertising and on advertising through sponsorship became greatly enhanced by powerful sections of the media and the sporting and cultural constituencies, resplendent with their high profile national celebrities, who often stood up publicly for their tobacco benefactors.

The tobacco industry had, for more than 16 years, financed massive advertising campaigns[2] urging that government leave the tobacco industry to advertise and sponsor in peace. As in other countries, it had established a well staffed and resourced and highly paid Tobacco Institute lobbying office. It had donated many millions of dollars over the years to political parties. Over this time, it had poured hundreds of millions of dollars into print media advertising and thereby compromised the editorial independence of the press in reporting and favourably commenting on initiatives to end this source of revenue.[3] And very significantly, the industry's business philosophy allowed it an affinity with the newly emerged, dominant political philosophies of free marketing.

Yet, in spite of all this, in a matter of only 16 years the Australian tobacco industry finally lost perhaps its most prized possession: the freedom to promote its products. The incremental victories of the Australian anti-smoking movement, which during this time culminated not only in the wholesale dismantling of a transnational industry's entire ability to promote its products freely, but the achievement of a one third fall in adult per capita cigarette consumption[4] will sit comfortably in the history of modern public health as one of the all time great victories.

The 1992 final curtain for tobacco advertising in Australia received support from all political parties, after a long history of strong opposition from the conservative (Liberal) opposition party. But what of the history that led to this historic decision? What agents of foment led to the social and political climate that eventually translated into a political majority supporting the vote? How was it, that, against all odds, relatively very powerless public health groups with few resources were able to win battle after battle against the economic and political clout of the tobacco industry?

Definition of public health advocacy

Similar questions can be asked of a great many modern public health initiatives that have been characterised by histories of public and political indifference or outright opposition; the existence of commercially and politically influential opponents; and public health proponents who are characteristically "amateur" in their resources. Recent international examples include campaigns to oppose the oil and automobile industries' resistance to removing lead from petrol;[5] the international movement against the Nestlé company's continuing promotion of breast milk substitutes, particularly in less developed countries;[6] and campaigns by Greenpeace and others against the dumping of radioactive toxic waste. One of the most notable and well publicised advocacy groups to emerge in the last decade is ACT UP (AIDS Coalition to Unleash Power), whose major achievements in the AIDS control field have been "to energize the fight against AIDS with an urgency that has translated into expedited drug approvals, lower prices for medications, and increased funding for AIDS research and care."[7] Membership of ACT UP has also allowed people with AIDS to resist the "passive patient" role and act against their stigmatised representation in the mass media and other public forums.

These are just a few examples of internationally known advocacy campaigns. But public health advocacy efforts are continually being undertaken at national, state, regional, and local levels too. A group of paediatricians who try to convince local and state governments to make domestic swimming pool fences compulsory to prevent backyard drownings; a group of residents who want their local government to erect more traffic calming speed humps and roundabouts to prevent children and old people being killed and injured; parents of children with allergies who want governments to ensure that grocery items are comprehensively labelled with information on food additives; women's health groups who try to have more women doctors and

5

nurse practitioners made available to take Papanicolaou smears; a group of school parents who want local shopkeepers to stop selling their children cigarettes. These are all examples of situations where the skills of advocacy can be essential to the objectives being sought.

Public health advocacy—sometimes called public health lobbying—is an expression used most often to refer to the process of overcoming major *structural* (as opposed to *individual* or behavioural) barriers to public health goals. Numbered among such barriers are some of the most formidable political, economic, and cultural forces imaginable. These forces include political philosophies that devalue health and quality of life at the expense of economic outcomes; political and bureaucratic opposition or inertia to health promoting legislative or regulatory provisions and policies, and to the participation of consumers in health care planning; the marketing of unsafe and unhealthy products, often by transnational corporations of immense influence and wealth; and the pervasiveness of major cultural values such as racism and sexism, which find expression in institutional values and personal attitudes and behaviours relevant to public health issues. The targets of advocacy then, can be the policies and practices of governments and large institutions whose actions affect the lives of many people; laws and government regulations; the commercial marketing practices of industries; and the activities of counter-health lobby groups who, if successful in their aims, can delay or obstruct the implementation of public health strategies such as universal health insurance, comprehensive immunisation programmes, fluoridated drinking water, compulsory front and rear seat belts, speed limits or cycle helmets.

Like all occupations, public health has evolved a specialist language which serves both to demarcate its professional territory and to express often complex and sometimes technical concepts. Around the mid-1980s, the word *advocacy* began to be used with increasing frequency in international public health circles. The word itself, of course, was not new. It had been used and understood for many years in the public health field by a disparate array of individuals and groups who tended to work on the fringe or completely outside of mainstream, government-sponsored public health projects. These were mostly single issue groups who had formed to advance their causes in the face of hostile, indifferent or non-existent government public health-related policies.

Before its recent renaissance, *advocacy* tended to have a rather confined use. It was a term used mostly to describe activity whereby representatives of the powerless, the oppressed, the poor, the disabled, and the sick would "advocate" for their rights. These representatives were either victims or sufferers of some affliction or injustice themselves, or else relatives, friends, or community members who spoke on the victims' behalf. Lawyers (who in many countries are actually called advocates), welfare workers, and church representatives were among those who typically engaged in advocacy on behalf of such groups. In the health care field, advocacy was generally understood to refer to the endeavour of promoting patients' rights and seeking to improve their access to services, entitlements and information. Indeed, computer searches of databases such as Medline still tend to locate research and commentary on this narrow definition of advocacy, limited to issues of patients' rights.

The recent embracing of the term by more mainstream public health interests appears to have gained momentum partly due to the influence of the World Health Organization's 1986 *Ottawa Charter for Health Promotion*, a document that has begun to permeate discourses about public health, both within the field and beyond it, in health administration and planning circles. The Charter describes seven broad strategies for building healthy public health policy, one of which is advocacy: "Political, economic, social, cultural, environmental, behavioural and biological factors can all favour health or be harmful to [good health]. Health promotion aims at making these conditions favourable *through advocacy* for health [our emphasis]."[8]

The term has rapidly become a buzzword, with its use becoming almost mandatory in any health politician's speech or major report. For example, the 1992 Report of the Royal College of Physicians of London, *Smoking and the young*,[9] emphasised the importance of advocacy in reorienting health services towards tobacco control goals. It recommended: "strengthen[ing] the public advocacy role of health professionals and health authorities [p85] and mobilis[ing] support and concern from parents, voluntary groups, local and national opinion formers [p82]."

7

But curiously, aside from such passing references and rhetorical flourishes to an allegedly central platform of public health strategy, there is very little that can be found that analyses or even describes the processes of public health advocacy or attempts to seriously instruct potential practitioners in its diverse skills. This book was conceived as an attempt to redress this gap. It is an attempt to examine both the *why* and the *how* of the ways that particular public health issues become prominent and politically compelling or actionable in an issue-rich political and news environment.

The upstream/downstream metaphor in public health

Public health advocacy is issue and policy oriented. It is not primarily oriented at changing the knowledge, attitudes, or behaviours of individuals, but rather the legislative, fiscal, physical, and social environments in which individual knowledge, attitude, and behaviour change takes place. There is a time honoured fable in public health which relates the analogy of a river, a cliff, and people who fall from the cliff into the river, as a way of comparing the impact and social status of clinical medicine with that of preventive health measures. The fable describes the expensive ambulances and the heroic rescue and resuscitation services that can be arranged along rivers to retrieve and revive those who are drowning. It acknowledges that those drowning are usually very grateful for these services and, conversely, that a lot of politically damaging fuss can be made if innocent or important people are left to drown.

As for the metaphorical cliff, the fable points out that safety fences erected at the top might prevent a lot of people from falling in. But it adds that fences can be ugly, that they disrupt views, and that as dull, static and unchanging objects they don't attract the same acumen as bright shiny ambulances or dramatic rescue routines. Above all, a fence does its job when *nothing* happens, while rescue services are frequently defined as successful when they are merely busy. The opening of a fence provides one photo opportunity for a politician; dramatic rescues can provide dozens.

Despite the obvious message of the fable (that there is common sense in erecting fences; that prevention is a wiser and more humane option than Sisyphean rescue, cure, and care services), there are many unfenced cliffs in public health and many others that topple under the slightest pressure. Yet fences such as advertising bans and restrictions, taxation policies linked to health objectives (for example, tobacco, alcohol, food, exercise, and sporting equipment), and policies requiring immunisation before school entry are examples of some of the most coveted goals in modern public health. This book is an exploration of this fable as it applies to the many and varied tasks that face public health workers. The book pays particular attention to the major factors that best help shape the social and political climates that ensure public health fences are built with enthusiasm and remain steadfast.

We emphasise throughout the book that the emergence of strong voices calling for change in public health policy and opposing those interests that stand in the way of optimum public health opportunities should not be seen as random, isolated events. Rather we hope to show that the processes whereby a public health issue comes to be defined as important by the public and key decision makers are amenable to both analysis and emulation.

Advocacy studies in academic purdah

Political decisions on health policies are occasionally taken by influential people of vision who lead their political colleagues to act without being spurred into action by mounting community pressure. More often though, governments are conservative and begin from the position of being more comfortable with doing little or nothing about public health issues, especially those strategies to control chronic disease, which (almost by definition) can be put off until another day. In the tobacco control field, for example, most of the important policy gains which have been made internationally have been achieved over decades through a great deal of advocacy and lobbying by dedicated individuals and associations, rather than through unexpected, serendipitous leadership from politicians.

As Carr-Gregg notes, governments tend to adopt policies only in a climate of public readiness, using the principle that governments should not move far from what is perceived to be public opinion.[10] The task for public health advocates is thus fundamentally involved with efforts to shift public opinion towards their preferred position, to the point where the desired political action becomes compelling, and inaction a political liability.

Most students of public health learn early of the consequences of John Snow's removal of the handle from London's Broad Street water pump, thereby stemming the city's cholera epidemic of the 1850s.[11] Snow's action is remembered for his epidemiological reasoning and its dramatic consequences more than for the tactics he employed or the opposition he faced in disengaging the pump. Yet without his direct and decisive action, the epidemiology would have mattered little and cholera would have continued to spread.

Although the point of this historical analogy may seem obvious, it remains curious that academic interest in *how* it is that the modern public health equivalents of Snow's actions succeed or fail in different social and political contexts tend to be marginalised as somehow unworthy of the name "research" or the critical gaze of scholarship. The main reasons for this appear to lie in the slippery and uncontrollable nature of the subject and in the awkwardness of the questions it intrinsically poses for the positivist research traditions that have hitherto dominated research in public health. Such questions though, can be of critical importance and can have profound consequences for the progress of public health policy implementation.

Consider the case, for example, of a government passing legislation to add fluoride to the water supply. Conclusions from a large and growing body of research in the epidemiological, dental health, and economic traditions are likely to have been fed to the politicians involved in the form of reports, letters, resolutions of support, and so on. Public opinion polls may have been conducted showing support for the proposed government action. Such studies provide currency to be used (and abused) by the parties to the debate in their efforts to argue their case. The traditional role of the researcher here is to address questions perceived to be critical to the evaluation of fluoridation and the likely consequences of its addition or removal, the assumption being that government policy will be research driven.

Yet only the most naïve would pretend that political decisions are always or even mostly determined in a way similar to that in which a piece of research might be scrutinised through a peer review process. The canons of scientific method allow research conclusions to be assessed against more or less agreed standards. By contrast, a political decision to add fluoride to the water supply may depend only peripherally on the quality and consistency of the evidence presented in its favour. Although such evidence is likely to be necessary to success in placing public health proposals on the political agenda, it is only rarely sufficient. The following factors are invariably also important yet remain in a research and analytic *purdah* in the mainstream public health literature.

The power of opposition groups

Many, although by no means all, public health issues feature struggles between proponents and opponents of particular proposals. Any public health policy or initiative that is not doggedly opposed by those vested interests that prefer the advantages brought by the status quo will almost certainly be of little consequence to the relevant public health objectives the initiative is intended to address. Thus any policy worth pursuing will be characterised by both overt and covert opposition that varies in strength throughout the world. The real or perceived power of opposition groups exemplified through direct or indirect financial support to politicians and their parties,[12] their ability to marshal equally powerful supportive constituencies in, for example, associated industries (such as, in the case of restricting tobacco advertising, in the advertising industry, agriculture, packaging, general retailing and small business, sport and culture), and their rating in national terms as economically important industries can be critical to the preparedness of governments or individual politicians to support public health initiatives.

Research examining the relationship between such power and policy success and failure is in its infancy. Outstanding questions include: has the power of opposition interests (or relative lack of it) been relevant in those countries that have successfully introduced particular public health policies? Have there been

11

tactics and strategies employed which have reduced or cancelled out aspects of an opposition's power in such countries? Is the effect of an opposition's power reduced if it is obliged to fight political battles on several fronts simultaneously? Are there manifestations of power which need to be nullified as preconditions to particular public health policies being taken seriously by politicians? For example, does tobacco sponsorship need to be replaced by government or alternative sponsorship before wholesale tobacco advertising bans will be seriously considered?

The framing of debate

There is no "objective reality" that any platform of public health policy can be said to be *really* about. To public health workers, compulsory bicycle helmets might mean reduced brain injury and deaths; to indifferent parents, their meaning might be framed more in terms of additional expense; and to fashion-conscious youths, they may well mean the intrusion of a paternalistic state on their ability to dress as they please and thumb their nose at danger. Reality is always a socially constructed notion.[13] The emphasis or framing that is placed around particular events or issues that seeks to define "what this issue is really about" will represent but one of many competing meanings that jostle for public dominance. Although health interests may frame the meaning of a bill to introduce fluoride to the water supply in terms of the protection of children's dental health, anti-fluoridationists may choose to describe the bill in terms of the encroachment of the "nanny state", "compulsory medication" and other negative metaphors.[2] Some questions here include: how best can these different framings be assessed in terms of their reception by politicians and others who make decisions about policies? Are there important differences in the framings favoured by those working in public health, and those that hold most public and political appeal? Are there methodologies that are sufficiently sensitive to be reliably used in pretesting different framings used in advocacy? What examples are there, where dominant framings that run against the interests of public health appear to have been successfully reversed? Are there principles that characterise such reversals, which can be applied in practical ways in future debates?

Pervasiveness of free market economic policy

The dominant international political and economic philosophy of the late twentieth century is free marketing. Margaret Thatcher's "pin-up" economist, Milton Friedman, one of the chief apostles of contemporary economic culture, once wrote: "Few trends could so thoroughly undermine the very foundations of our free society as the acceptance by corporate officials of a social responsibility other than to make as much money for their shareholders as possible."[14] Most supply-side policies in public health (for example, price policies, restrictions on ingredients, marketing restrictions, and safety standards) appear to derive from a different set of values. Where does this apparent disjunction leave political arguments to restrict certain activities of the free market known to have an impact on public health? To what extent have arguments about public health issues taken on any *exceptional* status within contexts of overall government economic policies on free markets? What framings and arguments have enabled this to happen?

Editorial coverage and conflict of interests

The mass media are essential to efforts to foment a social and political climate that is antipathetic towards destructive influences on public health such as smoking, drunk driving, and promoting social procedures and rules that work against violence or discrimination. Evidence continues to accumulate on the way that acceptance of tobacco advertising by the mass media is associated with reduced and sanitised coverage of tobacco and health and tobacco control issues.[15, 16] What effect has publicity about this relationship had on media owners and editorial staff, political decision makers and public opinion? What is known about the editorial processes involved in such circumstances? Are there other examples of latent or covert censorship of health issues through pressure from advertisers? Does "censorship" of pro-public health news and comment occur latently or overtly, and what implications does this hold for advocates? Can such censorship in particular media outlets be constructively sold as news value to others with more sympathetic editorial policies?

13

Public opinion

We live in an increasingly issue rich environment. Public health issues are concerns among many thousands about which citizens and politicians are invited to form opinions and to take actions. Little is understood about the relationship between changing public opinion and political action in public health. It is interesting to reflect on the nature of the occasions when public health issues become significant political issues for politicians and the public. How do politicians decide that single issues are worthy of the political spotlight? What do we know about the extent to which public health issues are voiced to politicians by their electoral constituents? Are such constituents seen as fringe or marginal by politicians? Is there a critical mass of voters that needs to be active before a politician senses that an issue needs to be taken seriously?

Political leadership

Key individuals within governments are often strongly identified with the passage of public health legislation. Little has been written other than the expected valedictory praise for such people. In circumstances where key individuals have been capable of influencing the political process *vis à vis* public health, what *actually* occurred to inspire their patronage? Are there generalisable lessons in such cases?

The political science of a political art

The knowledge that exists about these and many similar questions enjoys a paradoxical position in public health. Although there are few who would not acknowledge the importance of such questions, there are just as few who have devoted themselves to anything like a systematic approach to addressing them. The status of most of what is considered "good practice" in successful public health advocacy remains little more than oral history. When these histories are associated with particularly analytic and prolific individuals, such as California's Stan Glantz[17-19] or Britain's Des Wilson,[20] the lessons involved can receive wide circulation. But in many more cases, the passage of significant events are reported mostly in terms of the public relations glory of their simply having happened.

Those who move regularly between the two worlds of academic research and public health advocacy can attest that there is little incentive to try to combine the two in anything but a fleeting fashion. For example, a recent editorial[21] on the research agenda for "applied smoking research" failed even to allude to these sort of questions when calling for the strengthening and broadening of research. The major public health funding agencies in our own country have no categories on their application forms which remotely suggest that these issues might ever be addressed in legitimate, fundable research.

As yet, there is very little that could be called a political *science* of public health advocacy. Yet there is a great deal of acknowledged political *artistry* in this field, on both sides of the trenches. What are we to make of the shared intuition often acknowledged within our field about particular strategies being more or less valuable in advancing the political fortunes of public health? Or of particular individuals being "good" at advocacy? What are the precise questions that need to be asked about this more or less intuitive understanding of good practice, if we wish to pass forward lessons from past events? This book attempts to explore many of these questions.

This chapter opened with an example about legislation to end tobacco advertising. The day to day tactics, which eventually result in government policy shifts in the huge, vested interest arenas such as this example, can often seem unthinkable to the orthodox health worker. The tactics and strategies of advocacy and lobbying are not easily described in terms of "programmes". What is *done* in public health advocacy seldom lends itself to precise statement as an independent variable capable of direct replication by others. There are few definable steps amenable to the requirements of the "methods–results–discussion" format demanded by most public health journals, and which seem to define the boundaries of the acceptable. Papers on the "how to" of public health advocacy, either describing or analysing advocacy campaigns, are comparatively rare in the literature of public health. Notable exceptions appear among the references listed in this book. Courses on public health advocacy are taught in only a small handful of Master of Public Health courses around the

15

world. The teaching of health promotion and preventive strategies at postgraduate level in nearly all universities is dominated by "downstream" oriented issues such as individual and group behaviour change, patient education, and other strategies where individuals are the subject group of interest. Yet ironically, the record of advocacy in achieving "top down" preventive measures that impact on whole populations gives this activity an unparalleled importance.

Looking at the vast literature on health promotion programmes, it is almost as if there is, like Julian Tudor Hart's inverse care law of primary health,[22] an inverse analysis law operating in public health: the more trivial the intervention, the greater the research interest; while the greater the potential for population-wide effect, the scarcer the analysis.

Skills required in effective public health advocacy

In working towards changing public and political opinion in favour of, say, reduced vehicle speed limits, public health advocates need to adopt the same repertoire of opportunist, responsive, imaginative, flexible, dramatic, and above all newsworthy tactics that are the stuff of all successful public opinion, political, and commercial campaigning. Such tactics are rarely the *modus operandi* of bureaucratic government departments or of the quasi-experimental models of academic social science.

A skilled public health advocate should have competency in, and understanding of, a diverse range of subjects and roles. These include political science, the sociology of mass communications, the symbolic role of politics in the structuring of media and political discourses on health issues, and networking techniques. There are also many, very practical skills and issues that need to be understood concerning the way news media operate. These are just a few of what needs to be described as a continuously developing field of competence, where a sense of opportunism is indispensable to effective practice. This is a reflection of the implications that arise from new technologies, new products, new laws and regulations, and new oppositional strategy that characterise the landscape of the new public health. Accordingly, the contents of this book derive from an appropriately wide range of disciplines and influences. The book aims at providing both a comprehensive theoretical and research oriented approach to media analysis with a practical guide to ways of using theory and research to tackle media advocacy for public health issues. It should therefore be of interest not only to practitioners interested in conducting advocacy campaigns but also to those interested in media analysis of medical and public health issues.

Structure of the book

This book is divided into two parts. These may be said to be theory and principles (Part I) followed by practice (Part II). This is a crude division, with considerable overlap, because, as is often said, there is nothing so practical as a good theory. In the case of advocacy, the theory and principles that might be said to exist are almost entirely derived from the experiences of those who have been involved in campaigns to effect changes in legislation and other political decision making, resource allocation, commercial practices, and social policies. These campaigns have seldom been theory driven in any selfconscious way, with those active in the campaigns sometimes reflecting only in retrospect that in fact there was considerable method in what often seemed like journeys where they flew by the seat of their pants, using rat cunning and intuition more than following any predetermined, tried and tested pathways.

It will be clear from the title of the book and from practically every page that we regard the role of the news media as absolutely central to the conduct of public health advocacy. The conduct of public health advocacy does not *just* involve media advocacy, but in the mass society of the late twentieth century, the mass media are simply unparalleled as vehicles for setting public and political agenda about what is regarded as important and worthy of action. There are very few instances in the recent history of public health where advocacy staged through the news media has not played a pivotal role in effecting the changes sought by public health workers. Every staff member of a politician's office will attest to the high priority given to ensuring that politicians are fully informed about the news media's treatment of their portfolio and that every opportunity is taken to use the media to further political goals. The start to most working days in a political office involves reacting to or providing further information on a news item from the previous evening's television or that morning's press or radio. Reading the media logs from the night before is invariably the first and most urgent task.

The news media have an impressive record in directly influencing political and policy outcomes. Alan Otten, for 44 years a reporter for the Washington Bureau of *The Wall Street Journal*, writes, "Well done investigative reporting produces public outrage (or policy maker outrage) that forces new regulations and laws or tougher enforcement of existing ones. Ten-thousand-watt klieg lights turned on a situation focuses the minds of policy makers very fast."[23] George Lundberg, Editor of the *Journal of the American Medical Association*, believes, "In our society public media are irreplaceable as a mechanism for moving a problem to a solution."[23]

The cost of purchasing advertising time to inform and persuade decision makers or the public about the need for change in public health policy is mostly way beyond the means of most public health interest groups. In the USA, the traditional provision of free public service announcement (PSA) time is declining, and so the importance of media advocacy in allowing issues to be covered as news on television is thus growing.[24] Understanding the nature of news, especially what makes particular news about public health newsworthy, is an indispensable and core skill for anyone wishing to become a potent public health advocate. There are at least three main reasons for this.

Firstly, understanding the nature of newsworthiness can yield important insights into the development and reproduction of culturally dominant meanings put on health issues by the public. Where an advocacy group's objective is to win widespread public support and action for an issue, it is critical that it has a sophisticated understanding of existing, relevant, lay beliefs and attitudes and the relationship of these to the ways in which they are communicated through the news media. Being more attuned to the ways in which public health issues are framed by supportive or hostile media can be very instructive to the task of understanding how issues need to be reframed in order to steer public and political support in the desired directions.

18

Secondly, a solid awareness of the processes of newsgathering, reporting, and editing is vitally important in understanding political responsiveness, sensitivities, priorities, and funding decisions that are relevant to public health. Very often in public health, there are literally only a handful of key decision makers who need to be convinced to take a desired course of action. Such individuals, for example, politicians, senior bureaucrats, and heads of non-government organisations, are often highly sensitive to the ways in which the media are framing issues and setting public expectations about the roles they should perform. To become an astute observer and analyst of the news on public health is to take giant steps in the direction of thinking in the ways that preoccupy these decision makers: how to keep "good" news flowing about public health and how to turn bad news into good news.

Finally, a thorough understanding of news media cultures and their day to day practical routines and preoccupations is critical to the task of developing oneself into a potent and sought-after news source: into a person or organisation that helps make the news on public health, and not simply a person or organisation who jumps reactively to the agenda set in the media by others.

Part I of the book consists of four chapters. Following this introductory chapter, Chapter 2 begins with an overview of the international research evidence on the depiction of health issues in the news media, and on how this coverage has been consistently reported to be a major influence on public knowledge and perceptions of health issues. We then provide a brief review of some of the main ways that analysts of news media have approached their topic. These range from crude "hypodermic" effects models that are preoccupied with the overly simplistic question of: "What do media messages do to people?", to audience centred models which start with a quite different assumption ("What do audiences do with media messages?").

Common to both models is a consideration of the media messages or texts themselves. Here, the approaches of mass media researchers have ranged from the straightforward enumerative frequency counting of content analysis (showing, for example, how often stories on particular issues are reported), to more interpretive and culturally anchored approaches which seek to elucidate the deeper meanings of media discourses and

19

narratives: of how particular instances of news stories, for example, exemplify or re-tell ideologies and cultural mythologies which subtly direct audiences to consider the meaning of a health story in terms of its deeper, subtextual features. Public health advocates need to be thoroughly cognisant of this dimension to the debates in which they participate, rather than simply preoccupied by the overt or manifest content of the issues with which they are involved. We take a "constructionist" view of news formation. As explained by Gamson and Modigliani: "Media discourse can be conceived of as a set of interpretive packages that give meaning to an issue. At its core is a central organising idea, or *frame*, for making sense of relevant events, *suggesting what is at issue* . . . [our emphasis]." [25]

Chapter 2 also reviews concepts and principles of newsworthiness, addressing the basic question of "What makes a health story newsworthy?" This chapter considers how workers in news media select and construct news stories within the bureaucratic, organisational, and economic constraints of their workplace. It introduces the techniques of discourse analysis, examining the importance of topics, headlines, lead sentences, personalisation, visual material, quantification rhetoric, news actors, and news sources in conveying information and favouring certain viewpoints over others.

Chapter 3 applies the principles reviewed in Chapter 2. The range of recurring subtexts and discursive strategies that underlie news reports of public health and medical issues are illustrated through the use of case studies in reporting about public health which we have selected from 1993 television and press news reports from two countries (Australia and the United Kingdom). In the first part of the chapter we examine all the health reportage broadcast during an entire week on four Sydney television channels. We show that 80% of all health news stories broadcast during the week exemplified just four principal subtexts. These subtexts, we suggest, are what determined the newsworthiness of the items that were broadcast. We then consider further examples of newsworthy case studies from Australian and British press reports, showing how they were framed and detailing the elements that attracted the attention of the press.

Chapter 4 illustrates the relevance of framing to the study of the advocacy process. We provide two detailed case studies in public health media advocacy, both illustrating the principles of framing in action. The first describes a continuing struggle between health workers and a public lobby group in Australia over attempts by the health workers to have all private swimming pools adequately fenced to prevent children drowning. The second is a case study of the attempts of health workers and the tobacco industry to capture the dominant agenda over a proposal to ban sporting sponsorship by tobacco companies. These cases illustrate in detail how both advocacy groups and their adversaries have framed or reframed particular public health issues in attempts to advance (or retard) public health objectives.

Part II is the "how to" section of the book. It is arranged as an A–Z of advocacy strategy. We hope that this arrangement of what is a very diverse range of issues, tips and detailed discussion of advocacy strategies will prove to be as user friendly as possible. Des Wilson's 1984 book *Pressure: the A to Z of campaigning in Britain*[20] inspired this format.

References

1 Chapman S, Woodward S. Australian court decision on passive smoking upheld at appeal. *BMJ* 1993; **306**: 120–2.
2 Chapman S. Anatomy of a campaign: the attempt to defeat the NSW Tobacco Advertising Prohibition Bill 1991. *Tobacco Control* 1992; **1**: 50–6.
3 Chapman S. On not biting the hand that feeds you: tobacco advertising and editorial bias in Australian newspapers. *Med J Aust* 1984; **140**: 480–2.
4 Chapman S. Unravelling gossamer with boxing gloves: problems in explaining the decline in smoking. *BMJ* 1993; **307**: 429–32.
5 Wilson D. *The lead scandal. The fight to save children from damage by lead in petrol.* London: Heinemann, 1983.
6 Allain A. *IBFAN on the cutting edge.* Oslo: Dag Hammarskjold Foundation, 1991.
7 Wachter RM. AIDS, activism, and the politics of health. *N Engl J Med* 1992; **326**: 128–33.
8 The Ottawa Charter for Health Promotion. *Health Promotion* 1987; **1**: iii–v.
9 Royal College of Physicians of London. *Smoking and the young.* London: Royal College of Physicians of London, 1992.
10 Carr-Gregg M. Interaction of public policy advocacy and research in the passage of New Zealand's Smoke-free Environments Act 1990. *Addiction* 1993; **88** (suppl): 35–41S.

11 Snow J. *On the mode of communication of cholera*, 2nd ed. London: Churchill. Reproduced in *Snow on Cholera*. New York: Commonwealth Fund, 1936.

12 Begay ME, Glantz SA. *Political expenditures by the tobacco industry in California State politics*. Monograph Series. San Francisco: University of California Institute for Health Policy Studies; 1991: 55.

13 Berger P, Luckmann T. *The social construction of reality*. London: Allen Lane, 1967.

14 Friedman M, Friedman RD. *Capitalism and freedom*. Chicago: University of Chicago, 1962.

15 Warner KE, Goldenhar LM. The cigarette advertising broadcast ban and magazine coverage of smoking and health. *J Public Health Policy* 1989; **10**: 32–42.

16 Warner KE, Goldenhar LM, McLaughlin CG. Cigarette advertising and magazine coverage of the hazards of smoking. A statistical analysis. *N Engl J Med* 1992; **326**: 305–9.

17 Samuels B, Glantz SA. The politics of local tobacco control. *JAMA* 1991; **266**: 2110–17.

18 Samuels BE, Begay ME, Hazan AR, Glantz SA. Philip Morris' failed experiment in Pittsburg. *J Health Polit Policy Law* 1992; **17**: 329–51.

19 Begay ME, Traynor M, Glantz SA. The tobacco industry, state politics, and tobacco education in California. *Am J Public Health* 1993; **83**: 1214–21.

20 Wilson D. *Pressure: the A to Z of campaigning in Britain*. London: Heinemann, 1984.

21 Bauman KE. On the future of applied smoking research: Is it up in smoke? *Am J Public Health* 1992; **82**: 14–16.

22 Hart JT. The inverse care law. *Lancet* 1971; i: 405–12.

23 Otten AL. The influence of the mass media on health policy. *Health Affairs* 1992; Winter: 111–18.

24 Wallack L, Dorfman L. Health messages on television commercials. *Am J Health Promotion* 1992; **6**: 190–6.

25 Gamson WA, Modigliani A. Media discourse and public opinion on nuclear power. *Am J Sociol* 1989; **95**: 1–37.

2: Analysing news coverage

DEBORAH LUPTON

With the increase in government sponsored health promotion media campaigns in the 1980s, a growing body of public health literature has emerged dealing with the use and evaluation of mass communication in public health.[1][2] The academic study of mass cultural representations of public health, however, remains underdeveloped. This is especially so within public health communities where the news media are often seen as a "problem" rather than important forums for the discussion and interpretation of public health issues as well as a potential resource to be exploited by public health advocates and health promoters. The application of knowledge from such research to training in advocacy strategies is also very neglected. Yet the mass media, by definition, reach mass audiences, including key political and bureaucratic decision makers. If well informed about the processes of news reporting, public health advocates may be in the position of influencing journalists to report issues in ways more consonant with public health objectives. Awareness of the subtextual meanings and messages of news media accounts of health and illness, as well as their obvious topical content, is important in understanding the context in which lay health beliefs are formulated and expressed. Efforts at better understanding of principles of newsworthiness, of the framing of health issues in the news media, and of audience response hold great promise for upgrading public health advocates' understanding of news and other media processes.

Health promotion practice and evaluation often focus on

discrete, time limited and planned health advertising campaigns delivered through mass media, with the assumption that such campaigns are potentially important in influencing knowledge, attitudes, and behaviour germane to health. The coverage of health, illness, and health risk in the popular news media, however, represents a vast body of largely *unplanned* messages and information about public health issues. If a health or medical issue hits the headlines and prime-time television news, it often receives intense (and free) publicity. Sometimes such publicity is not supportive of public health goals. For example, media coverage of the few children who suffer adverse reactions to immunisation can act to distract from the importance of community-wide immunisation to prevent the emergence of epidemics of childhood diseases that once killed many. Big news stories on health regularly have a profound influence on public health policy, influencing public and political agenda, and community expectations. This coverage, generated as it is from the principles of newsworthiness, is often despite the public health importance of an issue.

Influence of health reporting

Owing to their popularity and position as the most "factual" and "important" element of the mass media, the news media often function as a lobby agency. As Nelkin[3] points out, "By creating public issues out of events, the press can force regulatory agencies to action simply out of concern for their public image." Nelkin asserts that it was newspaper publicity about toxic wastes dumped at Love Canal, New York State, which forced the New York State Department of Health to act, and which eventually brought about changes in national waste policy. Press coverage of laetrile as a drug used to treat cancer, and resultant public pressure, forced the (American) National Cancer Institute to test the drug on human cancer patients even though it had been shown to have no therapeutic effect on animals. The news media's attention to a health issue can also result in funding being made more easily available for research in that area.

Very few lay people read medical or public health journals, or policy statements, or attend scientific conferences. The news media are therefore vital in mediating between specialised forums for the dissemination of medical and public health research, and policy and the wider public. This is especially the case if a disease, condition, or health risk is unfamiliar, new, or rare. For example, by June 1983, virtually every American surveyed in public opinion polls had heard of or read about AIDS, even though only 3% of respondents reported actually knowing a person with HIV/AIDS.[4] News media coverage is integral in shaping public perceptions of risk, especially when people have little first-hand experience of an issue, or when the event is dramatic and unexpected, calling into question the practices of everyday life. In such a situation, "We turn to people with special insight into the hidden forces behind these events to help us better cope with the risks that we now suddenly recognise";[5] the news media provide such sources.

Population surveys repeatedly show that the mass media are nominated as the leading source of information about important health issues. Examples of such reports include those on dieting and weight control,[6] AIDS and HIV,[7–9] drug abuse,[10] asthma,[11] family planning,[12] and mammography.[13] In many countries, this reflects near-saturation levels of television and radio access, average weekly viewing hours that can rival time spent in the workplace and engaging in other forms of leisure combined, and the high circulation figures of popular magazines and news-papers. Watching television is the single most time-consuming leisure activity of Americans.[14] Senior American policy makers, including politicians and high-level public servants, also cite the news media as important sources of information about health and medical issues.[15]

Members of the public commonly express much interest in medical and public health news stories. For example, in a study of over 4000 adults in the United Kingdom and the United States, the highest level of self reported interest in categories of news stories was for new medical discoveries. When respondents were asked how likely it was that they would read newspaper stories under a variety of different headlines, medical stories were clearly in the lead, together with government expenditure cuts. It is worthy of note that only a few of those who reported a high level of interest in such issues felt that they were well informed about them. This lack of knowledge was revealed by the finding that when the respondents were asked if antibiotics are effective against viruses, only 28% of Britons and 25% of Americans were able to give the correct answer.[16] A study of American college students and their understanding of popular press reports of health research similarly found that, even among a relatively well educated sample, the overall rate of reader misunderstanding approached 40%.[17] The authors concluded that the public's inability to comprehend health information given in news articles may seriously flaw subsequent decision making about health risks.

Given its overall popularity as a medium of entertainment, television news is perhaps the most widely consumed forum for health and medical stories. An Australian journalism academic, John Henningham,[18] surveyed a random sample of people from Sydney, Melbourne, and Brisbane about television news in 1982. He found that 92% said they watched one or more television news programmes at least once a week. The level of interest in medical and health issues noted by Durant, Evans and Thomas in their American study[16] was reflected in Henningham's study: respondents said that they were most interested in news about scientific and medical developments and 78% said they had a high or very high interest in such news.

The power of the news media to place issues on the agenda for discussion has been demonstrated in the public response to medical controversies that have made headlines. In the early 1980s, the British news media reported the findings of a study published in a medical journal which revealed that pertussis (whooping cough) immunisation was associated with severe neurological illness in a small number of British children. As a result of media coverage, there was a dramatic fall in vaccine up-take in the United Kingdom, for which members of the medical profession blamed journalists.[19] Wellings[20] similarly found that there was a high degree of publicity accorded by the British press to the findings of two research papers published simultaneously in the *Lancet* suggesting a link between cancer and the oral contraceptive pill. She argues that the link with cancer and the simultaneous publication of the reports in the same prestigious journal incited the controversy. The response of family planning health professionals was to warn women "not to panic", a statement that made headlines and thus provided confusing messages for audiences.

Types of news media

When discussing the ways in which medicine and public health tend to be covered in the news media, it is also important to consider the differences between the types (or genre) of media that report news.

Television

Television has the largest reach of all mass media, combining both audio and visual stimuli in the viewer's own home. It covers health and medical issues in news and documentary programmes, commercial advertising, drama, cooking and sporting programmes, as well as screening government sponsored health promotion campaigns. One common problem with television is that the seductiveness of the visual image, while lending credibility (people can "see it for themselves") can often overwhelm the audio message. For example, although many people watch evening television news programmes, viewers often do other things while a programme is screening and thus do not give it their full attention. A 1992 study of the viewing habits of 1204 Australians found that 65% of people ate meals in front of the television and that only 34% admitted to giving their "full attention" to news programmes. Television was described in the report as a contemporary form of "aural wallpaper".[21]

The reliance of television news upon dramatic visual imagery means that, unless a story has good visual "grab", it is unlikely to make the news bulletin. Furthermore, as the average television news story is less than two minutes long, there is very little chance to present a complex issue in this medium. Newspaper coverage allows a more complete, and considered, account: it has been estimated that the total word content of a 30 minute television bulletin would only occupy about two columns of a broadsheet newspaper.[18]

27

Print media

These include newspapers, magazines, pamphlets, and books. Newspapers are an obvious constant source of information about health and medical issues, but many people read only selected items, or just scan the headlines rather than read a newspaper from cover to cover. There are major differences in the ways that the tabloid and the "quality", or broadsheet, press reports issues and events. In tabloid newspapers, huge headlines and large photographs take up some space at the expense of detailed discussion of news items, yet these newspapers are the most popular. News magazines such as *Time* and *Newsweek* provide detailed coverage, especially in their feature articles, which can run to several pages, but have a reasonably select readership. Women's magazines have high circulations, but often sensationalise or personalise issues. Such magazines, however, regularly feature informative articles on women's health issues such as breast cancer, pregnancy and childbirth, and sexuality. Self help books on health sell well, but there is no guarantee as to their quality or whether the reader reads the whole book or just sections.

Radio

Radio has a very wide reach, especially in the mornings and during "drive time" peak hours and among adolescents. There is a multitude of radio stations, however, each with a fairly narrow demographic audience. Furthermore, most people tend not to give radio their full attention—it is often background noise. Discussion and news programmes on some stations (often public radio or non-commercial radio such as the Australian Broadcasting Commission) provide excellent coverage of health and medical issues but have a comparatively small audience compared to commercial radio.

News values and the construction of news

There is a growing literature of content analysis studies of the frequency of the depiction of various health related issues, such as food,[22] [23] AIDS,[24] alcohol,[25] [26] oral health and dentistry,[27] tobacco advertising and its relationship to the frequency of press coverage of the hazards of smoking,[28–31] dementia,[32] tranquilliser use,[33] and abortion.[34] A study of the coverage of mental health topics in popular magazines between 1965 and 1988 found a significant increase in the number of articles and headings related to mental illness and treatment. The report focused on the finding that many of the changes in headings used were consistent with changes in the field—for example, the introduction of new diagnostic categories, and with desired changes in terminology, such as using less stigmatising terms.[35]

Much writing on health and the media springs from a priori expectations held by researchers of the roles, functions, and reporting criteria they seem to feel the media ought to fulfil.[36] One study, for example, examined the extent to which newspaper and magazine coverage of two risky situations (a nuclear power plant accident, and the relationship between coffee consumption and pancreatic cancer) included the kinds of "cognitive information" about risks that would help readers make informed risk judgements. Many press reports were found to be lacking in such information.[37] Another study reported how the media "distorted" public perceptions of psychiatric treatment outcomes involving sexual disorders and paraphilia. The authors concluded that inaccurate media presentations about psychiatric rehabilitation that ignore treatment successes and focus only on alleged failures do a "disservice to patients, mental health workers, and society at large".[38]

News as a social construction

Perspectives on news as a social construction argue that "news" is not the reporting of an objective reality, but a particular version of events, the end product of a series of selection processes based on a socially constructed set of categories and belief systems.[39] [40] To understand the ways in which news producers construct the news, news must be viewed as a product of a highly complex process of selection. Of all the myriad events that occur each day, only a tiny number are selected as "news". This selection is based on the unwritten laws and routines of newsmaking, and is confined within the organisational, economic and bureaucratic constraints under which newsgathering organisations operate: "News is not 'found' or even 'gathered' so much as made. It is a *creation* of the journalistic process, an artefact, a commodity even, as manufactured as a motor car or a Cruise missile; and in that manufacturing process strong forces exist to skew its content."[40]

In large newspapers, before a story is published, it is often handled by several individuals, including the chief reporter, a journalist, the subeditor, and the editor, most of whom may rework the copy more than once before it appears as a final product.[41] In television news, the news director, chief of staff, executive producer, correspondents and reporters, producers, subeditors, camera operators, and tape editors all have a hand to play in the production of news. The cyclical and cooperative nature of news production makes it difficult to identify who is the actual "author" of the text, especially as much of the material in the story may originate from a media release, previous news stories, transcripts of speeches, reports, agendas, minutes, and international news agency copy, audio-tape, or film.[41]

News for commercial organisations is a commodity, used to sell advertising space to industry in return for audience attention. As such, news must attract as many viewers/readers/listeners as possible, so that the maximum fee may be charged to advertisers. This dependence upon advertising revenue may have an influence on the type of news that reaches the public. In the quest for maximising profits, the wishes of advertisers are often taken into account when choices are made concerning news items. The revenue, for example, provided by tobacco manufacturers advertising in women's magazines in the United Kingdom and the United States was enough of an incentive to prevent those magazines from carrying articles describing the health risks associated with cigarette smoking. One study examined the coverage of tobacco hazards in 12 major women's magazines published in the United States between March 1967 and February 1979.[42] The researchers found a paucity of reporting on the adverse health effects of smoking in most magazines over that time, despite growing awareness in the community of the dangers of tobacco. In some cases, the dangers of smoking were even minimised or ignored in articles where such a discussion would have been appropriate. Those magazines that did run frequent articles on this topic, significantly, did not accept tobacco advertising, suggesting a direct link between the economic pressures applied by the tobacco industry to the print media.

Further evidence of the power wielded by advertisers upon the editorial decisions of the print media is provided by two studies of American magazines. One[43] reviewed the coverage of the health risks of smoking and drinking in *Ms*, an avowedly feminist magazine, during the years 1983 to 1986. The authors found that, although there was a significant presence of alcohol and cigarette advertising in the magazine, little space was devoted to the health risks associated with the use of these products. Advertisements for cigarettes and alcohol frequently invoked the socially desirable images of fitness, wealth and romance, and the challenging of traditional gender roles, but there was little in the editorial content of the magazine to challenge these images. In the second study, a number of popular magazines published between 1959 and 1986 were examined for their coverage of smoking and its health implications in the light of the cigarette broadcast advertising ban of 1971.[28] The study showed that, in the last year of broadcast advertising and the first year of the ban, cigarette advertising expenditure in magazines increased, while articles about the health risks of smoking in magazines that carried cigarette advertising decreased.

Principles of newsworthiness

Regardless of the medium (television, radio, or print) in which it is covered, the principles of newsworthiness include the following key criteria. "Good news" (that is, news worthy of coverage) includes the following elements:[44]

- New or unusual information
- An event that makes an impact
- A response to a current news event or statement
- The presence and statements of a prominent person
- A human interest story
- A bizarre or extraordinary person or event
- Closeness, occurring in the local region
- Drama, tragedy or having an effect on people's lives
- Evocation of an emotional response

- Conflict
- Elite or famous people or nations
- Ability to be personalised
- Part of an existing newsworthy theme
- Attribution to valued news sources
- Facts
- A scoop
- Statistics.

News and current affairs items are selected by television researchers, editors, and news controllers from an often vast array of potential items. These items vie for selection through presentation via national and international satellite services accessed by all television stations, through press releases, the activities of public relations firms, the choices made by journalists covering routine news beats such as politics, health, the courts, sport and business affairs, and by virtue of being deemed "hard" news—for example, major incidents, the activities of celebrities, and significant events such as elections and conflict.

The decision making processes through which items are both selected by journalists and editors for publication or broadcast, and framed through newsreader scripting, the selection and editing of interviewed persons and the use of film to illustrate the story have been much studied by media researchers. Much of this literature explores journalistic and editorial notions of news sense—that instinct journalists have, or claim to have, which tells them what is news and what is not, and how what is news should be presented. It has found that many decisions to select or reject news are made based on a system of unwritten rules about what is considered newsworthy or entertaining, what audiences expect or like, what will attract high ratings, what constitutes "good quality" or a "different perspective". These definitions are drawn from the ways in which media workers are acculturated as members of the general society in which they live, and more specifically, the manner in which they have learnt and become experienced at their profession:

A would-be radical journalist knows that he or she has to get copy past the sub-editor, and the television reporter faces similar shifting mechanisms of editorial control. He or she will know from bitter experience that "alternative" stories can be lost on an editor's desk, that they can be extensively rewritten on the way to the print room, or even that they can be tolerated this time at the cost of not having contracts renewed, or actually being sacked.[40]

However, it is not always the case that even highly experienced media workers can predict what makes a successful media product. An expensive television drama series, for example, which is screened with high hopes of it becoming acclaimed by critics and popular among viewers, may be greeted with widespread praise and receive high ratings, or it may sink like a stone and cease production.

Journalists' perspective

Health risks are particularly newsworthy when they involve human interest stories, personal dramas, dramatic research discoveries on dread diseases, disputes, and controversies.[45] Journalists must deal with complex scientific and medical data when writing about health risks but are constrained by the organisational aspects of their work to convey information simply, unambiguously, and dramatically, often resulting in certain relatively rare risks being exaggerated while others are minimised, and the omission of important details and sufficient critical analysis to allow readers to develop cogently notions of personal risk.[15-49] As a result, dramatic incidents that receive a high level of media coverage are more likely to be judged "risky" by audiences and readers than common, everyday hazards.[46]

Press reports of research articles published in the scientific and medical literature have been shown to amplify the subsequent citation of such articles in later scientific articles. A recent American report tested the hypothesis that researchers are more likely to cite papers that have been publicised in the popular press. They found that articles in the *New England Journal of Medicine* that were covered by the *New York Times* received a disproportionate number of scientific citations in each of the 10 years after the articles appeared. The effect was strongest in the first year after publication, when articles publicised by the *New York Times* received 72.8% more scientific citations than control articles.[50] There is evidence that newspapers will give greater attention to studies which report news of effectiveness (as opposed to no effect). Koren and Klein studied reportage of two studies on radiation and cancer risk, one negative and one positive, published back to back in a single issue of the *Journal of the American Medical Association* (20 March 1991). They found 17 newspapers in the United States which, between them, published 19 reports on the two studies. Nine reports were dedicated solely to the positive study and 10 reports covered both studies. None of the reports was dedicated to the negative study only. In reports covering both studies, the mean length of the positive reports was significantly longer than the mean length of the negative reports.[51]

As noted above, the news media tend to emphasise hazards that are relatively serious and relatively rare. One example is toxic shock syndrome, which emerged in the 1980s as a new disease related to the use of sanitary tampons, attracted a great deal of media attention for a time as an acute and potentially widespread illness, but has since failed to raise the interest of newsmakers. Singer and Endreny[47] assert that:

The media are superb at evoking the serious outcomes associated with a particular instance of a hazard—a specific car crash, nuclear reactor accident, death from toxic shock. But they fail to put such risks into perspective—not only the perspective of alternative hazards, which would be asking a good deal, but even the perspective of how likely such outcomes are; that is, the risk of their occurrence.

Kristiansen[52] undertook a content analysis of health information presented in over 1000 articles printed in seven British national newspapers over a three month period during the summer of 1981. She found that most articles about health were event rather than issue oriented, and gave only very superficial coverage. Information which might be useful for the audience, such as details about symptoms and preventive measures, was rarely mentioned, with the focus being on treatment, giving the impression that health status is beyond the individual's personal control. The quality newspapers devoted more attention to health issues and used more reliable sources of information than did the more popular newspapers. Attention was paid to rare illnesses and conditions, which account for few deaths, to the exclusion of more common causes of morbidity and mortality in the population. A content analysis undertaken of the coverage by the American press of cancer in 1977 and 1980[53] found that newspaper coverage lacked detailed information that would provide perspective on such a fear raising topic. News reports did not provide statistics on the incidence of cancer in general, and particularly underreported the recorded incidence of colorectal cancer relative to other types of cancer. Issues of prevention and detection received little attention. Most reports focused on three topics: causes of cancer, treatment, and famous people and cancer. About a third of all reports indicated that progress was being made in cancer research and treatment, and coverage tended to emphasise dying of the disease rather than coping with it. Fast-breaking events received most press attention, leading to coverage of cancer that was "fragmented and ephemeral".

While public health workers tend to criticise the bias, oversimplification or distortion they see in media reporting of health risks, they need to remember journalists' need to take information and represent it as an immediate, self-contained and easily understood news item. Many journalists who report on health and medicine do not have university degrees, let alone degrees in science, health, or medicine (although some of the élite newsmakers, such as the *Sydney Morning Herald* and the *New York Times*, do have medically qualified journalists on staff). These people, like journalists on other news rounds, must respond to the demands of their workplace, above all to newsworthiness. The imperatives of journalism rest upon drama, controversy, conflict, human interest, and brevity. As a result, the complexities of medical research or health risks are often simplified.[49] The constraints of limited space and the need to complete daily deadlines mean that journalists often do not have time to research exhaustively a news story on health and medicine. Journalists must deal with constantly changing events and scientific evidence, and present complex information in a way that will be readily understood by the audience. There is little time for detailed research into health issues, and therefore journalists tend to rely upon known sources of technical information, people or interested groups who are willing to give their opinion.[3] The journalistic convention of providing "both sides of the story" in the search for balance and fairness tends to rely upon established news sources, while ignoring other, less powerful individuals' opinions on the issues. When medical and health information is covered, conclusions are often inflated and their importance exaggerated. Issues are polarised, such that: "Even when responsible opinion on an issue is clustered in the centre, an otherwise unassailable journalistic account will sometimes provide 'balance' by juxtaposing the comments of quotable 'experts' whose views seem relatively extreme."[49]

It is frequently the case that findings of epidemiological research or medical trials are inconclusive and are not easily summarised in the news format. There has, for example, been a continuing debate in the medical and public health literature over the relative benefit of controlling serum cholesterol for individuals at risk of coronary heart disease. Given the level of dissent among scientists and researchers, it is not surprising that media reports have conveyed confusing messages about the risks of cholesterol. Even if the findings of medical or scientific research are inconclusive, equivocal, do not reach statistical significance, or are poorly designed, if they are published in a well respected journal such as the *British Medical Journal* or the *New England Journal of Medicine*, if the senior author of the article is well known, the subject is considered interesting to the readership, or the interpretations of the data are provocative, then the research will be deemed newsworthy.[49] One example is the coverage of an article in the *New England Journal of Medicine* which gave preliminary findings from a study investigating the preventive effects of taking aspirin regularly against heart disease.[54] Because the findings were contentious (rates of stroke were higher in the treatment group), the medical article stated that the public should not start taking aspirin to prevent heart disease. The five major American newspapers ignored this caution, however, and chose to champion aspirin taking, ignoring the greater risk of stroke associated with regular aspirin use. They also failed to discuss the strict requirements for entry into the study, which included the exclusion of participants who had a history of heart attack, stroke, cancer, or other conditions.

To summarise, news media's reporting of health and medical issues frequently displays the following characteristics:

36

- Regardless of degree of severity or prevalence, some health issues receive more media attention than others.
- The news media tend to distort information, favouring extreme views over more moderate, considered views.
- Therefore, health risks are often not placed in perspective against other risks of life.
- Media coverage of health risks and treatments is often contradictory and confusing for the audience—for example, immunisation might be reported in highly positive terms one week, then with suspicion the next.
- Coverage of risks gives a broad view, but often does not report on the reliability of the information used, give background information, or give more detailed information about the extent to which health risks might affect the audience.
- As a consequence, coverage of health risks tends to invite panic, but does not provide enough details to enable people to assess their own risk.
- Coverage often focuses on the dramatic nature of biomedical treatment rather than ways of preventing illness.
- The news media have the power to function as a lobby by setting public and political agendas on what is important and worthy of action.
- Commercial advertisers may influence the content of news stories about health risks.
- The source of the news story is important in determining the way in which the story is framed—for example, medical journal articles will tend to attract more legitimacy than the media releases of a consumer/activist group.
- Greater attention is given to health risks that are relatively serious and rare—for example, Legionnaires' disease and toxic shock syndrome—than to common, chronic health issues such as diabetes.

Analysing health and medical reporting

There are various methods used to analyse news media reports. The most commonly used method, traditional content analysis, focuses upon quantification of media content. Traditional content analysis dissects news texts—newspaper or magazine articles, transcripts of radio and television bulletins—into their smaller components, and then enumerates them. A researcher, for example, may be interested in tracing newspaper coverage of cancer over several years. After collecting all clippings from the newspapers included in the study, the researcher tallies the number of news items about cancer appearing in each different newspaper, the types of cancer (breast cancer, prostate cancer, skin cancer) mentioned in the articles and the means of treatment or prevention discussed in relation to cancer (diet, exercise, avoidance of sun exposure, surgery). These tallies can then be expressed statistically, and displayed as tables, graphs, et cetera. This method allows researchers to document patterns and trends in media coverage of health and medical issues over time, or to compare reporting in various different news media, or to compare coverage of some health issues with that of others. If, for example, a researcher was interested in comparing the level of news coverage accorded heart disease versus breast cancer, traditional content analysis provides an appropriate methodology.

Although quantification of news media content is an important way of tracing trends and patterns in coverage of medical and health issues, this technique is limited to documenting "what was said" rather than "how it was said". The number of times people are shown drinking alcohol on a television programme, for example, may be less significant in terms of the effect upon the audience than the attractiveness of the characters involved. To answer the second question, a complementary qualitative content analytical approach, discourse analysis, may be used to focus more closely on the language, images, and discourses drawn upon to create meaning in the media text. "Discourse" here is defined as a pattern of talking and writing about or visually representing an event, object, issue, individual or group. Discourses do not exist in a vacuum; they are sited within the historical and political contexts in which they are produced and reproduced and are understood by reference to these contexts. The wider belief systems giving meaning and structure to media texts are identified by this process of analysis. When analysing texts, discourse analysts are constantly asking such questions as: "Why was this said, and not that? Why these words, and where do the connotations of the words fit with different ways of talking about the world?"[55] The emphasis is upon identifying patterns, as well as discontinuities, in the texts. In taking this orientation, discourse analysis can assist in answering questions about who benefits and who suffers from the particular ways in which issues are reported or discussed in the media. Hence, discourse analysis comes from a critical perspective rather than a politically neutral one and is therefore an ideal method of media analysis for advocates.

Like other qualitative methodologies, discourse analysis is based upon interpretive skills, dependent on the individual analyst's sensitivity and insight. To be successful, the analysis must be conducted in concert with a wide knowledge of the sociological, historical, and political background of the news texts. The emphasis is not upon "proving" that the interpretation is "correct" or "accurate", as the method is not a positivist approach which assumes that "reality" is there, waiting to be discovered through scientific and objective processes. A high degree of selfconsciousness or *reflexivity* is therefore required in carrying out discourse analysis, incorporating an awareness that all knowledge is socially produced, that one is producing a discourse by analysing other discourses, that one is inevitably writing from a certain political position.

One study using discourse analysis examined the portrayal of the "salmonella in eggs" scare which occurred in the British press in the winter of 1988–9.[56] After the first press report that salmonella, a bacterium that causes food poisoning, had been found in eggs sold in Britain, the discourse of risk in the press escalated into a full scale hysteria. The headlines and main texts of the press reports incorporated a vocabulary of confusion, hazard, risk, danger, and crisis. Accounts suggested that the British public were being threatened by a very powerful and virulent enemy, and were rooted in the genre of horror stories and science fantasies about biological invasion and chemical warfare. The rhetoric of quantification was a major and dominant discursive strategy for inciting panic—the audience was bombarded with large numbers, all referring to different entities, populations, or time periods, creating an impression of confusion as well as danger. The use of verbs and nouns such as "increase", "rise", "grow", "spread", "leap" and "proliferation" contributed to this impression, as did the adjectives "astronomical", "sudden" and "rampant". Likewise, constant references to the words "poisoning", "health", "infection", "contamination", "pollution" and "hygiene" widened the issue and signified such meanings as anxiety, guilt, and ideas of responsibility, both public and private.

Another discourse analysis focused on newspaper coverage of tranquilliser dependence in British newspapers.[33] The authors noted that the news accounts concentrated on two kinds of tranquilliser users: the celebrity and the ordinary user, both of whom were usually represented as female. Such women were portrayed as passive "victims of circumstance", lacking control over their lives, biochemically addicted and helplessly controlled by the drug. They were represented as "innocent" drug users compared with the "guilty" users of illicit drugs such as heroin; their roles as respectable wives and mothers were emphasised to support their status as "innocent victims" of drug dependence. The tranquillisers to which they were addicted were personified as cunning, powerful villains, employing the metaphors of "drug as disease" and "drug as the devil".

Such studies reveal that health and medical news reports constantly draw upon discourses and ideologies that go beyond the narrow content base of the topic they are ostensibly discussing and tap into a range of concerns that preoccupy Western societies in the late twentieth century. News reports on health, medicine, and illness incorporate discourses associated with war, fear, violence, deviance, heroicism, gender roles, religion, xenophobia, contamination, vilification, control, and progress. They depend upon a series of binary oppositions such as male/female, us/them, self/other, normal/deviant, innocent/guilty, passive/active, hope/despair, and victim/villain to create meaning around these events and issues.

AIDS is a particularly vivid example of how media coverage of a health risk incorporates manifold discourses and ideologies that combine to form a web of meaning extending beyond the health risk to the fears of wider society. The discourses evident in the coverage of HIV/AIDS in the British, North American and Australian news media have tended to represent some people living with AIDS as "innocent victims" of the syndrome while others have been represented as "guilty", and blamed for their condition.[57-61] Negative responses to homosexuality, permissive sexuality, prostitution, and injecting drug use are reflected in this dichotomy. Media accounts of AIDS have frequently invoked the discourses of discrimination, prurience, racism and stigmatisation, and imagery associated with the plague, sin, deviance, divine retribution, leprosy, the apocalypse, and holocausts, all serving to create a sense of panic and emergency and incite vilification of people with or deemed at high risk of HIV infection.[61]

Health advocates need to be sensitive to these subtextual meanings in media accounts, for their very lack of obviousness enhances their unquestioning reception by audiences. It is vital for advocates to be able to understand the subtleties of such covert meanings, for successful advocacy depends upon recognising, discriminating, and constraining archetypes and ways of framing medical and public health issues, and then seeking to challenge them. Just as AIDS activists, for example, have publicly resisted the vilifying archetypes of the "innocent", non-gay person with AIDS versus the "guilty" gay man with AIDS, so other public health advocates need first to be aware of this type of representation, and then act to resist and reshape the archetypes.

Doing discourse analysis

As the above examples demonstrate, discourse analysis examines the choices of words, images and narratives used in media products, seeking to go beyond the obvious meaning to the subtextual layer of meaning. This section provides guidelines for advocates to undertake discourse analyses of the elements of news stories about their issue that combine to present a certain version of events.

Choice

A discursive process always involves choice in its construction, and the inclusion and absence of options are significant, going back to the social context: "Obviously journalists look for the dramatic and the sensational angle on stories, but the question is, *which* drama and *which* sensation to tell what kind of story?"[40] The choice of words is vital to the meaning of a

41

communication, demonstrating on which side speakers/writers are placing themselves; when referring to an embryo as a "fetus" or a "person", when describing people living with AIDS as "innocent" or "guilty", when calling a group of people a "mob" or a "crowd". For example, when anti-tobacco activists refer to cigarettes as chemical, carcinogenic cocktails they are constructing a discourse around smoking that refers explicitly to its link to death from conditions such as lung cancer and emphysema, and which combats the discourses of glamour, youth, physical activity, and vitality that tobacco companies use to advertise cigarettes. Each of the categories of news discourse below is dependent upon choices, which may be made either consciously, to achieve effects such as urgency, drama, conflict, and facticity, or subconsciously, as part of the general routine of gathering and producing newsworthy stories.

Topics

The topic of a news story is the specific event, issue, person, group, or thing that it refers to. A television news story reporting the outbreak of an epidemic of Legionnaires' disease, for example, is covering the topic "Legionnaires' disease". All topics, however, fit into one or more broader *topical themes*. A Legionnaires' disease outbreak story may fit into the topical theme of "epidemics" or "infectious disease". It is important to note which topics receive a higher level of coverage in the news media, as attention to particular topics over others is significant. For example, why is it that AIDS in the late 1980s received a very high level of media coverage, which has since subsided? Why is breast cancer, which kills more Australian women every day than people who die from AIDS in any year, deemed of less interest to audiences as indicated by the far fewer news items devoted to this disease?[62]

The answers to these questions must consider political issues, which then relate back to *subtextual themes*. Subtextual themes are those that are not immediately obvious, but which link the topic to wider sociopolitical discourses. They therefore go beyond the topic to examine the ideological context in which they "make sense". As noted above, for example, AIDS has been commonly linked with the discourses of homophobia, sin, deviance, and divine retribution. The media have frequently drawn upon these in the attempt to attract audience interest and to understand the phenomenon in ways that draw upon dominant shared understandings and assumptions that are already established. Thus the notion that male homosexual sexual activities are "wrong" and "unnatural", and that gay men are "Them" and not "Us" seems to fit in well with the advent of this new disease, which in Western countries has affected gay men more than others. By using these wider discourses, media workers frame the issue in certain ways, attempting to direct audiences towards their preferred understanding. That is not to say, of course, that all audience members will be receptive or positive towards such attempts at meaning production—a point that is elaborated upon in detail later in this chapter.

Headlines

Headlines are an important feature of newspaper reports, as they are conspicuous, printed in large, bold type, are designed to attract the attention of the reader, and are often the only part of the news story that the reader will read. They are somewhat less prominent in broadcast news, but are often found at the very beginning or end of the news bulletin, summarising the main stories of the day. Because of their prominence and their function in summarising the main topic of the story, headlines signal to the reader how to "define" the situation or event reported.[63]

Headlines are a specific genre of news writing that eschews the conventions of the orthodox sentence by presenting the crux of the news story in as few words as possible in the attempt to attract readers' attention and invite them to read on. Headlines are far shorter than most orthodox sentences, commonly consist solely of nouns and verbs, with fewer articles, clauses, conjunctions, and adjectives than orthodox sentences and little use of punctuation. This simplified structure does not mean that headlines are dull; on the contrary, the careful selection of nouns and verbs, the use of common rhetorical devices such as alliteration, punning, metaphors, references to other genres and discourses, and the creative use of a restricted lexicon mean that headlines are fascinating parts of news language.

One example is the headline "MOW THE LAWN AND DROP DEAD"

that appeared on the front page of one of Australia's most prestigious broadsheets, the *Sydney Morning Herald* (16 November 1992). The story was reporting a study published in the *Medical Journal of Australia* that week by two pathologists who had come across five cases of men who had died from severe coronary arteriosclerosis, having suddenly collapsed while mowing the lawn at home. The article went on to note that strenuous physical activity contributes to cardiac attacks for men with heart disease (surely not a new discovery). This story made the front page of the *Sydney Morning Herald* because the subeditor who wrote the headline was able to dramatise the report by emphasising the potentially fatal nature of a banal domestic activity carried out by thousands of their readers on a regular basis. In just six words the headline simplified the main newsworthy properties of the story—the combination of death and everyday activities—in a way that suggested an inevitable cause and effect chain (implying that anyone who mows their lawn could suddenly lose their life). The headline arouses curiosity, inciting readers to read on and discover the reason for this surprising statement. There was probably more than one newspaper reader that day who vowed to use the risk of sudden death as an excuse not to mow the lawn the following weekend!

Lead sentences

Lead sentences are the second most important feature of a newspaper report, as they follow the headline and serve a similar function in summarising the most important aspects of the news story as perceived by the journalist. As Bell[41] notes, "The lead is a micro-story. It compresses the values and expertise of journalism into one sentence. Understanding how the lead works is to understand the nature of news stories." All news stories are written in the "inverted pyramid" format: that is, they begin with the information deemed most important and interesting, and end with that considered least important. The first one or two sentences need to detail "who", "what", "where" and "when". The reason for this structure is that stories often have to be edited down for space or time reasons, and the first parts of the story to go are the end sentences. The equivalent in the electronic media is the first sentence uttered by the news announcer for each individual news story in the bulletin. Subeditors usually rely on the journalist's first few sentences to construct the headline, so the tenor of these sentences will often shape that of the headline.

In the article about the health hazards of mowing lawns discussed above, for example, the lead sentences were: "Science has finally come to the support of all those men who complain at weekends that mowing the lawn can be a killer. Perth pathologists who investigated the cases of five men who died while cutting their grass have warned about the potentially strenuous nature of the activity." The first lead sentence begins on a light, somewhat frivolous note, punning on the phrase "can be a killer". The second is more serious, bringing in the "expert" news sources and noting their warning about the ill effects of mowing. The headline picked up on the frivolous tenor but also emphasised the dramatic nature of the second sentence.

News sources and actors

When considering persuasion in news accounts, it is important to examine from whose perspective the topic is discussed, whose opinions achieve prominence and which news "actors" and news sources are drawn upon. Virtually all news stories feature at least one news source or actor, whether an individual, an organisation or group, or an article published in a medical journal. In a study that I conducted of front page news stories on health and medicine published in the *Sydney Morning Herald*[64] it was found that less than 3% of these stories had no news actor or source, with a mean average of 3.8 news actors or sources per story overall. Other studies which have examined the use of news sources in medical and public health stories have found that government officials, medical journals and "celebrity" authorities receive the greatest coverage.[37 65 66] Shepherd,[65] for example, found that in reporting issues concerning marijuana use, those news actors receiving most attention from the American press were government officials, not scientists or physicians engaged in relevant research projects. Rather than citing medical studies concerning marijuana, news stories relied upon statements made by "celebrity" authorities to whom expert scientific or medical credentials were imputed.

45

As these findings suggest, news sources and news actors in medical and public health reporting are not always chosen for their scientific or medical knowledge or expertise in a particular area, but for their public position, renown or fame. Often, direct quotes from news actors or news sources constitute the news in their own right. The choice of "talking heads" can thus determine the way in which events are interpreted by audiences and readers of news accounts, setting the agenda for discussion of an issue and on occasion influencing government policy. The more famous the news source or actor, the more likely this is to happen. People whose opinions regularly make the news are politicians, officials, celebrities, sports people, and criminals. "Ordinary" individuals and the disadvantaged tend to be ignored by the news media unless they commit a crime or are involved in an accident or are witnesses to crimes or accidents.[41]

My own study of front page news[64] found that, in medical and public health stories, patients and advocacy groups trailed élite groups such as politicians and government officials, researchers/academics, and the medical profession in succeeding in having their opinions sought by journalists for important stories. I also found a striking gender imbalance in news sources and actors: almost three quarters were male. Linked to this finding is the fact that established sources, politicians, officials, academics—people in positions of power—are easy for journalists to contact and give legitimacy to a news story. The more authoritative a person's title (President, Prime Minister, Professor, Minister of Health), the more prestigious their affiliation, the more likely it is that their comments will appear. This means that members of élite groups in society have their opinions reproduced in news stories far more than the person in the street, and that men, who continue to hold positions of power in greater numbers than women, will dominate as news actors and sources. One political consequence of the use of élite sources is that journalists tend to suppress critiques of that person or their organisation, so as not to jeopardise their chances of using that source again.

An example of the importance of news sources and actors is the media attention drawn towards AIDS issues when it is revealed that a well known person has HIV infection or has died of a condition related to AIDS. In most Western countries, it was not until the famous Hollywood actor Rock Hudson became ill from

AIDS related illnesses in late 1985 that the news media devoted much attention to the AIDS epidemic, even though, since 1981, thousands of people had died of the syndrome. Indeed, neither President Reagan nor Vice-President Bush referred to the AIDS crisis in their country until 1987, even though their positions would have done much to enhance awareness of the syndrome among Americans. Gay spokespeople were quoted on the American network news far less frequently than non-gay authoritative news sources such as politicians or doctors.[4] When American basketball player Ervin "Magic" Johnson revealed at a media conference that he was HIV positive in 1991, intense media interest (even in Australia) surrounded his announcement because of his status as a highly paid and extremely popular sports figure in the United States. Johnson maintained that he had contracted the virus through heterosexual sexual activities, and thus served to draw attention to that route of transmission. By the end of the day in which Johnson held the press conference, the American National AIDS Hotline had received over 10 times the usual number of AIDS related inquiries.[67]

Such *personalisation* of news features is a common strategy of reporting, used to encapsulate and render more immediate the major issues by providing an illustrative case study. Personalisation of news issues is how many "ordinary" people make the news. If there is an outbreak of infectious disease in an area, for example, journalists often seek out someone who has fallen ill, or their relatives, to interview. Such a case study is especially newsworthy if the ill individual has been saved from death or permanent disability by the medical team and is extremely grateful, or conversely, if he or she believes they have been treated badly or negligently, and wishes to complain or even sue the authorities involved. And the more famous the person involved, the more likely it is that they will be chosen to "personalise" the disease or condition involved.

Photographs and other visual material

As mentioned earlier in this chapter, television news is far more dependent upon striking visual images than the print media, and an issue or event will rarely make the television news if there are not images to accompany it—the more dramatic and visually compelling, the better. Although the print news media are not quite as dependent on images as television, many news stories are accompanied by photographs or other images, such as graphs, charts or maps. This is especially the case if the news story is on the front page of a newspaper, as this section of virtually all newspapers features at least one large photograph. News magazines are similarly reliant on colourful photographs, graphs, or other visual images to illustrate their stories.

When analysing media coverage, it is important to pay attention to the choice of visual images, noting the communication of meaning therein. Whose faces or bodies are shown (and whose are absent)? How are they shown in relation to each other? What do the photograph captions say? What symbols and signifiers are used to convey meaning, to denote status, authority, passivity, or other meanings? What meaning systems are drawn upon to allow audiences to "make sense" of the imagery? If the images are in colour, what colours are used, and what meanings do they convey? What is the background (context) of the image? How are statistics represented in graphs and tables, and to what purposes?

A large black and white photograph, for example, used to illustrate a story on an outbreak of Legionnaires' disease in an area of Sydney printed on the front page of the *Sydney Morning Herald* (24 April 1992) depicted a scene from a hospital emergency room. Two male doctors (recognisable by their gowns and surgical masks) and a female nurse (also wearing a surgical gown) were shown clustered around a bed, on which lay a faceless patient, seemingly unconscious and recognisable as male only by the visible, hefty forearms emerging from the bed covers. The paraphernalia signifying "hospital"—wires, tubes, machines—to which the patient was attached surrounded the bed. One doctor was shown holding the patient's head, and both doctors were looking intently at the nurse, who was grimacing and had her hand to her forehead in a gesture signifying distress. Given the context, the distress appeared to be caused by the stress of the influx of sudden cases of Legionnaires' disease into that hospital. The general air was one of emergency being dealt with by medical expertise. This "reading" of the photograph is supported by the headline above the photograph—"Frank battles a killer he thought was just flu"—and the caption "Liverpool

48

Hospital's Dr Adam Purden, Dr Richard Maynard and Sister Cathie Jacks attend a legionnaire's patient". It is notable that, while the headline implies that the patient is actively "battling" the virus, the photograph depicts a passive patient, helplessly confined to bed while the forces of medical expertise bustle around on his behalf.

Close attention to the use of numbers, statistics, tables, and graphs is important to understand the rhetorical importance of such devices—for example, a study of the use of graphs to represent the drug use in American print media found that the graphs frequently misrepresented the extent of the problem to achieve visual relevance and drama and to suggest an "epidemic" of drug use among American students.[68] Even though rises in percentage terms may have been relatively slight—as little as less than 2%—the graphical representation of this rise implied a major change and impending crisis, supported by headings such as "A COKE PLAGUE" and subheadings such as "Within the next two years, more than 20% of high-school seniors may have tried cocaine."[68] Thematic logos also have important rhetorical power: for example, "THE DRUG CRISIS" used to head news stories published in *Newsweek* about drug use for several years, or the image from the Australian "Grim Reaper" AIDS education campaign in 1987, which used a horror movie icon of the symbol of death, and which was adopted by several newspapers to head any article about AIDS published during that year.[61]

Analysis of audience response

While it is important that advocates are aware of the properties of news and how the discursive features of news stories convey meaning, it is also desirable that they have a sophisticated understanding of how members of the audience respond to such representations. Early research into mass communication grew out of models of personal communication, which focused upon the effectiveness of a message as it passed between sender and receiver. This model of communication has been called the stimulus–response or "hypodermic syringe" model, because it viewed audiences as virtual *tabula rasa*, uncritical absorbers of media messages. Just as a hypodermic needle injects a drug into a patient with the expectation of an effect to follow, media messages were seen as "doses" of influence which could be expected to "affect" all those who were exposed. This perspective still crops up today, especially in regard to debates about the effects of sex and violence depicted on television. It is sometimes evident in health promotion literature on the use of the mass media, in which it is often assumed that a media education campaign will have the power, single-handedly, to change health related behaviours. It is now recognised that such an approach is far too simplistic.

A sociology of mass communications later developed, moving away from the idea of a passive audience to the concept of a highly active, highly selective, and "obstinate" audience, manipulating rather than being manipulated by mass media.[69] Audiences were classified by their tastes for media, their socio-demographic characteristics, their beliefs and attitudes and personality traits. This approach has been called the "uses and gratifications" perspective. Research adopting this perspective focused on the uses audiences made of the material they consume from the media, the influence of social groups upon the reception of messages, the ways that media texts were produced and the effect of "gatekeepers", such as newspaper editors, in mediating messages.

From the late 1960s, and gaining dominance in Europe and Australia in the 1970s, the British cultural studies approach to the study of communication also began to challenge the traditional "effects" approaches to studying media. Cultural studies theorists began to inquire into the social context in which media messages are both constructed and received. Researchers began to study how people used the mass media during the routine of their everyday lives; for example, how they discussed television programmes or used news items or the latest travails of "soap opera" characters in conversations with friends. Using this perspective, the newspaper may be regarded not only as a source of reporting on the day's events, but as "a linking mechanism between the rituals of the domestic, the organisation of the schedule of everyday life and the construction of the 'imagined community' of the nation", while watching evening television news similarly may be conceptualised as participating in "a joint ritual with millions of others", regardless of the information content of the actual newspaper or broadcast.[70]

Rather than viewing media products as having highly structured meaning systems, which enforce a particular version of reality upon audience members, it was recognised that audience members vary in the ways they interpret media. As a result, media products are said to be polysemous, or having many (rather than a single) possible meanings, and audience members may be viewed as having different "subject positions" which are ever-changeable. Depending on such sociodemographic factors as an audience member's gender, ethnicity, social class, age, education background, occupation, sexual orientation, nationality, and personal experience of the issues involved, the intended meaning of the message may be accepted, negotiated, or resisted.[71] Although it is accepted that people rely on established knowledge and belief systems in making sense of media messages, and that audience members often share a cultural repertoire, the cultural studies approach argues that there is the potential for variability within this repertoire.

A television news item, for example, championing the benefits of radical mastectomy for women with breast cancer, perhaps including an interview with a patient who has recovered successfully after this treatment, may be regarded by some viewers as evidence of the progression and beneficence of modern medicine. A woman viewing, who has been diagnosed with cancer and awaiting similar treatment, may well find such a report reassuring and credible. These subject positions readily accept the "preferred" meaning of the report—the meaning intended by those who have put the news item together. If, however, another viewer has known a close family member who recently died from breast cancer after undergoing a mastectomy, accompanied by side effects, he or she may feel more cynical about the claims of the treatment as portrayed in the media report. Alternatively, a viewer who is perhaps a trained nurse who has cared for many patients with breast cancer may have mixed feelings about such a report, given her or his experience in seeing the variable outcomes of mastectomy. Such responses for each position are changeable, depending on the context in which they are assumed. As Morley[70] comments, "We can see the person actively producing meaning from the restricted range of cultural resources to which his or her structural position has allowed access."

It is also recognised, however, that there are limits to the different ways in which media texts can be "read". The producers of such texts as news accounts invite and attempt to persuade audiences to arrive at certain "preferred" meanings through the language and wider discourses they use to frame issues. Media texts are produced from a pool of common discourses and meanings and are read within that framework of possible meanings.[63][72] By referring to certain discourses and narratives, the producers attempt to provide signposts as to how they prefer audiences to read the text: "While the message is not an object with one real meaning, there are within it signifying mechanisms which promote certain meanings, even one privileged meaning, and suppress others: these are the directive closures encoded in the message."[70]

The choices made by the producers of the text, the presence of some signs and the absence of others, are vital here. The weight of control is clearly in the hands of the producers, writers, editors, and journalists involved in constructing a news story. They decide which words and images to use, which sound bites or grabs are used and which are left on the cutting room floor, and who is asked to speak on an issue in the first place—for example, those individuals routinely requested by journalists to provide quotes for their news stories, tend, as I have discussed above, to be drawn from certain social categories. Even if Ms Brown from the suburbs has a strongly held opinion on a health issue, her view will generally not be sought by journalists unless she is a "victim" or good material for a personalised news story, such as the mother of a child who has the illness in question. Even then, the portrayal of Ms Brown will emphasise, not the "expert" nature of her views, but her status as an "ordinary" person and "mother". She may be interviewed at length, but her statements will be edited to possibly a four second bite for the television news and she will not have any control over which of her words are chosen for this purpose.

Contemporary audience studies typically examine differences between the reception of media messages by different subcultural groups. Kitzinger and Miller recently adopted this approach to investigate the impact of news accounts of AIDS upon British audiences.[73] They showed prerecorded excerpts from British television news programmes to various socially diverse groups from Scotland and England, including medical practitioners, male and female sex workers, prisoners, police officers, school students, retired people, and office cleaners. In a focus group session, the groups discussed the television extracts and also were asked to write collectively their own news bulletin using a set of photographs taken from television news footage. Kitzinger and Miller[73] found that audience groups tended to display cynicism and distrust about the news media's coverage of AIDS issues, but also demonstrated that they had received many of their ideas about AIDS from this source. The authors suggest that people tend to accept more readily media messages that fit into a broader context which has already been established in their knowledge of the world. For example, individuals were more likely to accept that Africa is "the source and hot-bed of HIV infection" because this fits with notions of Africa as the "dark continent", a "death zone" of deprivation, dirt, promiscuity, and contagion. Under such an understanding, it "makes sense" that AIDS originated and proliferated in Africa. Conversely, personal experience, position in the class order, ethnicity, understanding of racism, or experience of oppression encouraged some people to be critical of media representations of African AIDS, although not invariably.

Conclusion

For the public health advocate, awareness of the political and ideological dimensions of media coverage of health and medical issues, and sensitivity to the ways in which language and discourse are vital in constructing versions of reality, are integral steps towards achieving greater insight into the sociocultural dimensions of health, disease, and medicine. Relations, structures, and practices of power are often taken for granted, routine and subtle. Discourse analysis, if undertaken from a critical perspective, serves to focus attention upon the exercise of power of social élites and the ways in which social inequality is reproduced, making them more obvious. Critical discourse analysis, therefore, because it is concerned not simply with the manifest, or obvious, content of text and talk, but also seeks to display the reproduction of ideology, and the more subtle forms of control, persuasion, and manipulation in the meanings inherent in discourse, both popular and arcane, is an ideal academic method for activist and advocacy activities.

By exposing the social and political bases of medicine, health care and illness, by showing how they are not necessarily given or "true" but are subject to change, by calling attention to the power relations inevitably involved, discourse analysis helps to render these phenomena amenable to negotiation, alternative ways of thinking and therefore the opportunity for resistance or subversion on the part of advocates for change. Importantly, an awareness of the political nature of discourse also enables health promotion practitioners and advocates to become aware of their own use of language, their own assumptions and practices, their "ways of knowing" and the competing interests involved in their work.

References

1 Wallack LM. Mass media campaigns: the odds against finding behaviour change. *Health Educ Q* 1981; **8**: 209–60.

2 Flora JA, Wallack L. Health promotion and mass media use: translating research into practice. *Health Educ Res* 1990; **5**: 73–80.

3 Nelkin D. *Selling science: how the press covers science and technology.* New York: WH Freeman, 1987: 82.

4 Colby DC, Cook TE. Epidemics and agendas: the politics of nightly news coverage of AIDS. *J Health Polit Policy Law* 1991; **16**: 215–49.

5 Stallings RA. Media discourse and the social construction of risk. *Soc Problems* 1990; **37**: 80–95.

6 Crawford DA, Worsley A. Dieting and slimming practices of South Australian women. *Med J Aust* 1988; **148**: 325–7, 330–1.

7 Dolan R, Corber S, Zacour R. A survey of knowledge and attitudes with regard to AIDS among grade 7 and 8 students in Ottawa-Carleton. *Can J Public Health* 1990; **81**: 135–8.

8 Robb H, Beltran ED, Katz D, Foxman B. Sociodemographic factors associated with AIDS knowledge in a random sample of university students. *Public Health Nurs* 1991; **8**: 113–18.

9 Chang HG, Murphy D, Diferdinando GT Jr, Morse DL. Assessment of AIDS knowledge in selected New York State sexually transmitted disease clinics. *N Y State J Med* 1990; **90**: 126–8.

10 Wright JD, Pearl L. Knowledge and experience of young people regarding drug abuse, 1969–89. *BMJ* 1990; **300**: 99–103.

11 Brook U. An assessment of asthmatic knowledge of school teachers. *J Asthma* 1990; **27**: 159–64.

12 Adamchak DJ, Mbizvo MT. Family planning information sources and media exposure among Zimbabwean men. *Stud Fam Plann* 1991; **22**: 326–31.

13 Baines CJ, Christen A, Simard A, Wall C, Dean D, Duncan L. The National Breast Screening Study: pre-recruitment sources of awareness in participants. *Can J Public Health* 1989; **80**: 221–5.

14 Kubey R, Csikszentmihalyi. *Television and the quality of life: how viewing shapes everyday experiences*. Hillsdale, NJ: Lawrence Erlbaum Associates. 1990:69–107.

15 Weiss CH. What America's leaders read. *Public Opinion Q* 1974; **38**: 1–21.

16 Durant JR, Evans GA, Thomas GP. The public understanding of science. *Nature* 1989; **340**: 11–14.

17 Yeaton WH, Smith D, Rogers K. Evaluating understanding of popular press reports of health research. *Health Educ Q* 1990; **17**: 223–34.

18 Henningham J. *Looking at television news*. Melbourne: Longman Cheshire, 1988: 16, 131.

19 Karpf A. *Doctoring the media: the reporting of health and medicine*. London: Routledge, 1988: 168.

20 Wellings K. Help or hype: An analysis of media coverage of the 1983 'pill scare'. In: Leathar D, Hastings GB, O'Reilly K, Davies JK, editors. *Health education and the media II*. Oxford: Pergamon, 1985.

21 Zuel B. The rise of the switched-on, tuned-out TV viewer. *Sydney Morning Herald* 1993 Feb 11; 3.

22 Story M, Faulkner P. The prime time diet: a content analysis of eating behavior and food messages in television program content and commercials. *Am J Public Health* 1990; **80**: 738–40.

23 Morton H. Television food advertising: a challenge for the new public health in Australia. *Community Health Stud* 1990; **14**: 153–61.

24 Pitts M, Jackson H. Press coverage of AIDS in Zimbabwe: a five-year review. *AIDS Care* 1993; **5**: 223–30.

25 Wallack L, Grube JW, Madden PA, Breed W. Portrayals of alcohol on prime-time television. *J Stud Alcohol* 1990; **51**: 428–37.

26 Breed W, Wallack L, Grube JW. Alcohol advertising in college newspapers: a 7-year follow-up. *J Am Coll Health* 1990; **38**: 255–62.

27 Noguerol B, Follana M, Sicilia A, Sanz M. Analysis of oral health information in the Spanish mass media. *Community Dent Oral Epidemiol* 1992; **20**: 15–19.

28 Warner KE, Goldenhar LM. The cigarette advertising broadcast ban and magazine coverage of smoking and health. *J Public Health Policy* 1989; **10**: 32–42.

29 Amos A, Bostock Y. Policy on cigarette advertising and coverage of smoking and health in European women's magazines. *BMJ* 1992; **304**: 99–101.

30 Amos A, Jacobson B, White P. Cigarette advertising policy and coverage of smoking and health in British women's magazines. *Lancet* 1991; **337**: 93–6.

31 Warner KE, Goldenhar LM, McLaughlin CG. Cigarette advertising and

magazine coverage of the hazards of smoking. A statistical analysis. *N Engl J Med* 1992; **326**: 305–9.

32 Commissaris CJ, Jolles J, Visser AP. 'Dementia' and 'memory' in daily and weekly publications: an analysis of newspaper clippings in the period 1987–1990. *Tijdschr Gerontol Geriatr* 1991; **22**: 21–7.

33 Gabe J, Gustafsson U, Bury M. Mediating illness: newspaper coverage of tranquilliser dependence. *Sociol Health Illness* 1991; **13**: 332–53.

34 Infante-Castaneda C, Cobos-Pons Y. Induced abortion in figures: analysis of the dissemination of statistics in the press. *Salud Publica Mex* 1989; **31**: 385–93.

35 Wahl OF, Kaye AL. Mental illness topics in popular periodicals. *Community Ment Health J* 1992; **28**: 21–8.

36 Oxman AD, Guyatt GH, Cook DJ, Jaeschke R, Heddle N, Keller J. An index of scientific quality for health reports in the lay press. *J Clin Epidemiol* 1993; **46**: 987–1001.

37 Ryan M, Dunwoody S, Tankard J. Risk information for public consumption: print media coverage of two risky situations. *Health Educ Q* 1991; **18**: 375–90.

38 Berlin FS, Malin HM. Media distortion of the public's perception of recidivism and psychiatric rehabilitation. *Am J Psychiatry* 1991; **148**: 1572–6.

39 Hall S, Critchter C, Jefferson T, Clarke J, Roberts B. *Policing the crisis. Mugging, the state, and law and order.* London: Macmillan, 1978: 53.

40 Philo G. Bias in the media. In: Coates D, Johnston G, editors. *Socialist arguments.* Oxford: Martin Robertson, 1983: 130–45.

41 Bell A. *The language of news in the media.* London: Basil Blackwell, 1991:34–5, 41, 176, 194.

42 Whelan EM, Sheridan MJ, Meister KA, Mosher BA. Analysis of coverage of tobacco hazards in women's magazines. *J Public Health Policy* 1981; **2**: 28–35.

43 Minkler M, Wallack L, Madden P. Alcohol and cigarette advertising in Ms magazine. *J Public Health Policy* 1987; **8**: 164–79.

44 Galtung J, Ruge M. Structuring and selecting news. In: Cohen S, Young J, editors. *The manufacture of news: social problems, deviance and mass media.* London: Constable, 1973:62–72.

45 Nelkin D. Communicating technological risk: the social construction of risk perception. *Ann Rev Public Health* 1989; **10**: 95–113.

46 Short JF. The social fabric at risk: toward the social transformation of risk analysis. *Am Sociol Rev* 1984; **49**: 711–25.

47 Singer E, Endreny P. Reporting hazards: their benefits and costs. *J Commun* 1987; **37**: 10–26.

48 Greenberg MR, Sachsman DB, Sandman PM. Risk, drama and geography in coverage of environmental risk by network TV. *Journalism Q* 1989; **66**: 267–76.

49 Klaidman S. How well the media report health risk. *Daedalus* 1990; Fall: 119–32.

50 Phillips DP, Kanter EJ, Bednarczyk B, Tastad PL. Importance of the lay press in the transmission of medical knowledge to the scientific community. *N Engl J Med* 1991; **325**: 1180–3.

51 Koren G, Klein N. Bias against negative studies in newspaper reports of medical research. *JAMA* 1991; **266**: 1824–6.

52 Kristiansen CM. The British press's coverage of health: an antagonistic force. *Media Inform Aust* 1988; **47**: 56–60.

53 Freimuth VS, Greenberg RH, DeWitt J, Romano RM. Covering cancer: newspapers and the public interest. *J Commun* 1984; **34**: 62–73.

54 Molitor F. Accuracy in science news reporting by newspapers: the case for aspirin for the prevention of heart attacks. *Health Commun* 1993; **5**: 209–224.

55 Parker I. *Discourse dynamics: critical analysis for social and individual psychology*. London: Routledge, 1992: 3–5.

56 Fowler R. *Language in the news*. London: Routledge, 1991.

57 Watney S. People's perceptions of the risk of AIDS and the role of the mass media. *Health Educ J* 1987; **46**: 62–5.

58 Watney S. *Policing desire: pornography, AIDS and the media*. London: Comedia, 1987.

59 Treichler PA. AIDS, homophobia, and biomedical discourse: an epidemic of signification. In: Crimp D, editor. *AIDS: cultural analysis, cultural activism*. Cambridge, MA: MIT, 1989: 31–70.

60 Patton C. *Inventing AIDS*. London: Routledge, 1990.

61 Lupton D. *Moral threats and dangerous desires: AIDS in the news media*. London: Taylor and Francis, 1994.

62 Lupton D, Chapman S, Wong WL. Back to complacency: AIDS in the Australian press, March-September 1990. *Health Educ Res Theory Practice* 1993; **8**: 17.

63 van Dijk TA. *Racism and the press*. London: Routledge, 1991: 50–1.

64 Lupton D. Medical and health stories on the *Herald*'s front page. *Aust J Commun* (in press).

65 Shepherd RJ. Selectivity of sources reporting the marijuana controversy. *J. Commun.* 1981; **31**: 129–37.

66 Greenberg M, Wartenberg D. Newspaper coverage of cancer clusters. *Health Educ Q* 1991; **18**: 363–74.

67 Brown WJ, Basil MD. Impact of the 'Magic Johnson' news story on prevention. Paper presented to 33rd International Communication Association Conference, Washington DC, May 1993.

68 Orcutt JD, Turner JB. Shocking numbers and graphic accounts: quantified images of drug problems in the print media. *Soc Problems* 1993; **40**: 190–206.

69 Bauer R. The obstinate audience. *Am Psychol* 1964; **19**: 319–28.

70 Morley D. *Television, audiences and cultural studies*. London: Routledge, 1992: 21, 136, 268.

71 Hall S. Encoding/decoding. In: Hall S, Hobson D, Lowe A, Willis P, editors. *Culture, media and language*. London: Hutchinson, 1980: 128–38.

72 Fiske J. *Introduction to communication studies*. London: Routledge, 1990:164 5.

73 Kitzinger J, Miller D. *In black and white: a preliminary report on the role of the media in audience understandings of 'African AIDS'*. Glasgow: AIDS Media Research Project, 1991: 11, 20.

3: Two studies of public health news

DEBORAH LUPTON AND SIMON CHAPMAN

As we have stressed so far in this book, a vital part of developing potent public health media advocacy skills is to have a thorough understanding of the concept of newsworthiness. Public health advocates often wonder why their preoccupations are not deemed interesting or newsworthy by the media. The simple answer is that advocates frequently fail to cast their stories within frames that are compatible with traditions of news. In this chapter, we will move back from a direct concern with media advocacy and explore how public health and medical stories are covered by the media. Our intent here is to illustrate both the scope of news reporting on health and to explore what ingredients seem to be required to make a health or medical story "big". The techniques of discourse analysis of media content explained in Chapter 2 will be used to examine a series of selected themes and topics from news media in Australia and the United Kingdom.

This chapter is based on two studies we undertook in 1993 of news coverage of health and medical issues. In the first part of the chapter, we review a full week's health news coverage by all Sydney television stations in March 1993, a month chosen at random. We then turn to the print news media and explore examples of press reportage of health stories in both Australia and the United Kingdom during that same month, with particular emphasis on the news stories that either received a particularly high level of coverage or were related to advocacy activities. The case studies address in detail the question "What made these stories newsworthy?" by examining the news actors and sources, the headlines and main texts, the subtextual narratives and metaphors, and the apparent news values that framed or carried each story.

Freaks, moral tales, medical marvels, and Grandma's advice: the newsworthiness of health in a week of Australian television

During the randomly selected week spanning 15–21 March 1993, we videorecorded the prime time evening news bulletins on Sydney television channels 2 (ABC), 9, 7, and 10, as well as all four evening current affairs programmes shown on these channels (*The 7.30 Report, Real Life, A Current Affair*, and *Hinch* respectively). All items, with the exception of sport, finance news, weather, "coming up next", reviews of "tonight's top stories", newsreader sign-offs, advertisements and programme promotions, were categorised under 17 headings based on categories used in previous studies of Australian television news.[12]

Table I shows that there were 432 news and current affairs stories broadcast during the seven nights, on 27 news bulletins and 20 current affairs programmes. The high ranking of politics may have been inflated due to the sample week falling immediately after the 1993 Australian federal elections when election post mortems and profiles of the victors and the vanquished abounded. Health and medical stories ranked equal third out of the 17 categories. This ranking would have been higher if the definition of the health category had included many of the trauma stories classified in the "accidents, fires and misadventures" category; some of the loss of life stories counted in the "disasters, storms" category; several stories on air quality that were placed in the "environment, nature" category; and several fund raising stories about health facilities that were placed in "events, openings, anniversaries, fund drives". The decision was made, however, to conform to categories previously established by other studies of Australian television news,[12] so these stories were categorised accordingly.

There were 24 different health and medical stories which,

Table I: News categories in seven days of Sydney television news and current affairs programmes

Category	Items (%)
Politics	73 (17.0)
Crime, courts, police	57 (13.3)
Medicine, health, science	37 (8.6)
Light, quirky, human interest	37 (8.6)
Accidents, fires, misadventures	35 (8.2)
Economy, industry, agriculture	30 (7.0)
War	23 (5.4)
Entertainment	23 (5.4)
Demonstrations, protests	22 (5.1)
Famous people	21 (4.9)
Major disasters, storms	16 (3.7)
Social issues, problems	13 (3.0)
Environment, nature	10 (2.3)
Events, openings, anniversaries, fund drives	10 (2.3)
Corruption	9 (2.1)
Culture, fashion, history	8 (1.9)
Ordinary people's achievements	5 (1.2)
Total	429

given some repetition of topics across channels, were broadcast 37 times (Table II). Of the 24 items, only five were considered sufficiently newsworthy to be broadcast on more than one bulletin or programme. Outstanding among these was a story about a local politician's call for smoking to be banned in hotels and clubs. This issue was covered on nine bulletins, three times more than the next highest ranked item, the famine in southern Sudan where, according to the story "800 000 people are starving to death". Nearly a third (12 of 32) of the health items were of overseas origin, an identical proportion to the overseas origin of all news items (sport excluded).

We found that 23 of the 24 different stories could be readily categorised as instances of at least one of four main narrative subtexts (Table III). Each of these subtexts is now discussed in detail.

Table II: Health/medical stories in one week of Sydney television news and current affairs programmes

Topics	Frequency
Move to ban smoking in NSW hotels and clubs	9
Famine in the Sudan	3
Doctors may be sued for failing to diagnose HIV	2
Researchers discover gene for breast cancer	2
Soldier contracts HIV in Cambodia	2
Improved drinking water for western Sydney area	1
16 year old girl with progeria	1
Anabolic steroid use in gymnasia	1
Irish Siamese twins separated	1
AIDS epidemic in Thailand	1
Aspirin prevents cancers of digestive tract	1
Former cancer sufferer helps Royal Women's Hospital	1
HIV infected doctors	1
Cervical cancer test to replace Papanicolaou test	1
Mother and son have heart–lung transplant	1
Drop in cot death in Australia (sleeping position)	1
New strains of 'flu coming	1
Heavy menstruation treatment	1
Doctors face litigation *re* childbirth	1
Obesity clinic at local Sydney Hospital	1
New cosmetic surgery fat removal treatment	1
New blood washing technique for reducing cholesterol	1
Study shows eating carrots and oranges will reduce coronary heart disease	1
Careflight brings sick child from Vanuatu for medical care	1
Total	37

The bizarre

As the quintessential visual medium, television tends to use only those stories that provide a vehicle for images that make compelling viewing. Hence, it is not surprising that every news item broadcast in this study was accompanied by film footage. Indeed, a number of topics that occupied the screen during the

Table III: Major narrative themes of health and medicine news stories

---

The bizarre:
  Famine in southern Sudan
  16 year old girl with progeria
  Anabolic steroid use in gyms
  Irish Siamese twins separated
  Obesity clinic at local Sydney hospital
  New cosmetic surgery technique for fat removal

Moral tales and falls from grace:
  Soldier contracts HIV in Cambodia
  Anabolic steroid use in gymnasia
  HIV infected doctors
  AIDS epidemic in Thailand
  Doctors may be sued for failing to diagnose HIV
  Doctors face litigation *re* childbirth
  Former cancer sufferer helps Royal Women's Hospital
  Careflight brings sick child from Vanuatu for medical care

Medical miracles:
  Researchers may have discovered a gene for breast cancer
  New cervical cancer test
  New treatment for heavy menstruation
  Obesity clinic at local Sydney hospital
  New cosmetic surgery technique for fat removal
  New blood washing technique for reducing cholesterol
  Mother and son have heart–lung transplant
  Irish Siamese twins separated

Low tech prevention:
  Move to ban smoking in hotels and clubs
  Drop in cot death in Australia due to change in sleeping position
  Study shows eating carrots, oranges will reduce coronary heart disease
  Aspirin prevents cancers of the digestive tract
  Improved drinking water for western Sydney area

---

sample week might not have been considered newsworthy if they had not featured strong visual imagery. This is especially true of those six news stories we categorised as "bizarre" items, which all featured film of bodies *in extremis*: the very fat and thin, the grossly muscled, and people with rare medical conditions.

The three Sudanese famine items, for example (on ABC and Channels 10 and 7's news bulletins on 16 March 1993), all used the same footage showing naked or semi-naked emaciated villagers, with intriguing warnings such as "We warn that some scenes in this report from Southern Sudan are disturbing".

An item on anabolic steroid use featured on Channel 7's news bulletin (15 March) was portentously labelled a "special report" and featured shots of heavily muscled men and women dressed in skimpy Lycra outfits exercising in gymnasia, tantalisingly and pointedly described by the reporter as "the singles bars of the '90s". This story held the news advantages of being both a bizarre story and a moral tale. It was introduced by the newsreader with the words that the drugs "offer a short-cut to massive muscles and a great-looking corpse", while an interviewed steroid user confessed that "gym junkies want to look good without the hard work". The use of the word "junkies" in this context denotes deviance and lack of self control as well as the laziness implied in the phrases "short-cut" and "want to look good without the hard work". A medical professor, given the last word in the item, described bodybuilders who use steroids as "fools". These words evoke the core lessons of the ascetic protestant ethic that life's rewards must properly be preceded by pain, hard work and denial, and that pride for many comes before a fall.

The Siamese twins separation item screened on Channel 9's *A Current Affair* on the same evening was patently a freak of nature story. Early this century, Siamese twins were paraded before the public in circus and freak shows. With public sensibilities now preventing such open voyeurism, the attempts of modern medicine to right the wrongs of nature conveniently allow the same public curiosity to be satisfied via an unquestioning and self justifying veneration of the surgical skill involved. In a lengthy sequence lasting more than half the allotted 30 minutes' screening time, viewers were shown many close-ups of the young Irish girls involved, their parents consulting with doctors concerning their surgical separation, and articulating their hopes and fears about the impending surgery, and interviews with the parents following the death of one of the girls soon after the surgery.

The item screened on Channel 7's news bulletin on 15 March on the community birthday party celebration for "the oldest little girl in the world"—a 16 year old Australian girl with progeria (Hutchinson–Gilford syndrome)—was an exemplary instance of the way in which television can masquerade the active pandering to a community appetite for freak show voyeurism as a legitimate news story. Progeria is a rare genetic disease with striking features that resemble accelerated aging.[3] It is so rare that, in 1990, only one case had ever been reported in China, the world's most populous country.[4] The "news" here was that the girl was having a birthday—an event that happens to everyone once a year. The birthday provided a pretext for the news programmers to allow viewers to gawp at a bizarre medical condition, with any hint of insensitivity being mitigated through the well-wishing of the newsreader and the implication that viewers had almost been invited guests at the girl's party. The reporter announced that those attending the party were said to have "guarded the secret of little Becky Coss for 11 years", thus inviting viewers to feel that the secret was being divulged then and there, a device that was extended to close the item coyly and with tasteless irony:

Reporter: But at sweet 16, Becky Coss is keeping one wish a secret.
Adult at party: You're sweet 16 and never been kissed before. What do you say to that?
Becky: Yes and no!

Moral tales and falls from grace

Six stories were based on subtexts that told moral tales about the dangers of self indulgence, the wages of sin, or medical negligence. The "gym junkies" item (see above) was an overt moral tale about the dire health consequences of narcissism; three items about HIV in Thailand and Cambodia warned about the dangers of visiting prostitutes in Asia (screened on *Hinch*, Channel 10, 15 March and 19 March, and Channel 10 news, 19 March); and an item about an HIV positive British gynaecologist was framed in terms of moral outrage about a conspiracy of silence to protect diseased, deviant doctors at the alleged expense of the health of thousands of ordinary women (*Real Life*, 16 March). In the Channel 10 news item describing the case of an Australian soldier who returned from Cambodia infected with HIV after having had sex with a prostitute, the alleged transmission incident was described as "a spur of the moment encounter with a prostitute after a few beers on a day off", thus defining the circumstances of transmission as an aberrant "straying from the path of righteousness" by a man portrayed in every other respect as normal and decent (it was emphasised in the report that "The soldier is a married man, one of more than 100 in the Australian communications team sent to Cambodia as our contribution to the UN peacekeeping force"). The probability of such a single episode of intercourse leading to female-to-male HIV transmission is extremely remote[5] but this consideration went unchallenged in the item's concern to depict the man's case as one of the folly of "boys being boys". The victim-blaming moral discourse of the item was also explicit, however: as one reporter commented, "It's not as if the army failed to educate the soldiers sent to Cambodia. It even supplied protection". This case provided television with a cautionary tale concerning the health effects of lack of adherence to safer sex guidelines yet, interestingly enough, failed to question the soldier's decision to engage in marital infidelity with a sex worker. There was also an element of xenophobia in the story, with the mythical "Far East" being depicted as a hot-bed of infection and disease, with statistics on galloping HIV infection accompanying film of outdoor markets and crowd scenes of Asian people.

Doctors featured as news actors in all but three of the 24 different health and medical stories screened during the sampled week. In the great majority of these, doctors played roles as heroes, technicians, experts, or sages (research boffins making discoveries and breakthroughs, skilled body sculptors, clinicians, and harbingers of warnings). In three instances, however, the news value of the stories lay in the portrayal of doctors as having fallen from their usual venerated position. Two stories concerned medical negligence: the potential for doctors to be sued over childbirth incidents (ABC news, 17 March) and for failure to detect HIV (Channels 7 and 10 news, 15 March). The third story was a lengthy report from the United Kingdom which was screened on *Real Life* (Channel 7) on 16 March, concerning a gynaecologist who was HIV positive. The item was introduced by Stan Grant, *Real Life*'s presenter, with the following words:

It's the best kept secret in Australian medicine—the numbers of doctors infected with the AIDS virus, but still treating patients. Now the official view is that the known risks of passing on the virus are small, so why add to the patients' worries? But that view is under increasing attack, as you can understand, especially after a recent case in England of a gynaecologist who'd treated thousands of unsuspecting women.

The reporter then set the stage for a conspiracy story by asserting that "Doctors infected with the AIDS virus and thousands of their patients kept in the dark unless they find out by chance" and repeating the main story frame immediately after her first comment: "Medicine's best kept secret. But should it be?" Two of these "unsuspecting" patients were then interviewed, articulating their dread, shame and fear: "I can't go out now. I come home, and that's it. I've stayed indoors. I won't go out. You know, I'm just being treated like a leper."

The suggestion was that even though the patients had tested negative for HIV, they were stigmatised by mere association with the seropositive doctor from whom they had received treatment. The news interest of this story was in the inversion of the stereotype of the person with HIV/AIDS as posing a threat to health workers and medical professionals, in concert with the discourses of conflict, secrecy and medical negligence. Doctors were represented as endangering their patients' lives and refusing to acknowledge it, casting into doubt their status as altruistic carers (we discuss these issues in more detail below, in our analysis of the British press's coverage of the same news story).

The story on a former cancer sufferer who was helping a hospital with fund raising shown on *Hinch* (16 March) was also essentially a moral tale, although one intended to evoke admiration and emulation, rather than the assessments of blame, guilt, or caution evinced in the other items in this category. So too, the item on the Australian Careflight transport of a sick child from the south Pacific island of Vanuatu to an Australian hospital drew on the moral discourses of Australia's benevolence and caring to sick and ailing children from less "fortunate" countries. The personalisation of the sick child directed viewers to consider that in the mass of starving, sick, and war-torn children who frequently fill foreign news items on television bulletins, Australian authorities were ready to be compassionate towards an individual whose anonymity and chances of imminent death were thereby transformed, fairy tale fashion, into a child with a name, a history and a future. This subtext is one with which most viewers would be very familiar, being common, for example, in the regular news items about the effects of Australia's international aid efforts and in charity appeals to help the peoples of famine-stricken countries.

Medical miracles

There were eight events that could be categorised under the subtextual theme of "medical miracles". The emphasis in these stories was on glorifying the "breakthrough" and success of medical science in its battle against human disease and death. The terms "world first" and "new" appeared several times in these stories, in concert with stock footage of medical and nursing staff clustered around a patient in an operating theatre, close-ups of electronic monitoring machines, and interviews with doctors in their emblematic white coats, all icons signifying medical progress and efficiency as a scientific discipline.

During the sample week the *Hinch* current affairs programme featured a story on an Australian mother and son who had both undergone heart–lung transplants (17 March). This was especially newsworthy not only because both had survived the operation and appeared to be healthy, but because they were the first known mother and son who had both undergone such a procedure, and because the son's heart had been donated to a third person. As presenter Derryn Hinch introduced the story: "An Australian mother and her son, suffering from the same heart and lung problems, now have a second lease on life . . . along the way, they've also helped another life be saved."

Both mother and son, referred to as "marvels of modern medicine", were quoted as saying that their lives had improved immeasurably since the operation: "To be alive, it's really great to be able to walk around and not be on oxygen and not be in a wheelchair . . . It's really something that I didn't expect I'd be able to do."

To emphasise their new-found robustness, mother and son were shown engaging in light physical exercise: gingerly cycling on exercise bicycles, sitting side-by-side doing bicep curls with a tiny weight, and walking on the beach. To add to the miraculous element of the story, a third patient was introduced: a woman who had received the son's discarded heart after his transplant.

Other such stories included the discovery of a gene believed to predispose women to developing breast cancer (Channels 7 and 10 news, 16 March), a test for cervical cancer (ABC news, 17 March), new treatment for heavy menstruation (ABC news, 18 March), the obesity clinic at Royal Prince Alfred Hospital (Channel 7 news, 17 March), a cosmetic surgical technique for fat removal (*Real Life*, 19 March) and a "blood washing" technique for reducing serum cholesterol (Channel 9 news, 19 March), as well as the previously discussed item on the separation of Siamese twins screened on *Hinch*. Only once (in the last-mentioned story) were the drawbacks or side effects of the surgical technique involved discussed at any length, and this only because one of the separated twins died following the surgery. The portrayal of the other "breakthroughs" tended towards obfuscating the socioeconomic and political reasons for ill health or conditions such as obesity, and neglected discussion of the alternative means of dealing with obesity or high cholesterol levels that are directed at prevention rather than costly and invasive medical treatment. The story on a trial procedure described as "blood washing", for example, framed the technique as a one-off miracle cure for the weak willed. The story positioned the technology as science's alternative solution to the dreary asceticism and denial involved in selecting a healthy diet and completely avoided any consideration of broader questions about the food selection, marketing, and distribution environment that encourages people to eat diets rich in fat.

Low tech prevention

Only five news items described recent research findings that pronounced the folk remedy wisdoms of yore to be beneficial to health. These items stood in contrast to the medical miracle items in that, although the second valorised science's ability to improve on nature (surgical fat removal, improved host resistance through blood washing) or science-as-detective (gene for breast cancer found, new cervical cancer test), the first showed that science, in all its complexity, often was humbled in the face of common sense: eating vegetables is good for you (Channel 9 news, 19 March); the mysteries of cot death lie in a baby's sleeping position (Channel 9 news, 18 March); regular use of inexpensive aspirin, obtainable over the counter at pharmacies or supermarkets, may protect against cancers of the digestive tract (Channel 10 news, 16 March); and ensuring clean water supplies prevents ill health (Channel 7 news, 15 March).

The discourse underlying each of these stories is that of the resilience of simple lay wisdoms about health in a world of scientific progress moving faster than many viewers could comprehend. Part of the power and appeal of this discourse derives from the intertextual referencing of such simple truths against the frequent honouring of the new in medicine. For example, as a postscript to the blood washing story described above, a brief item on an American Heart Association study claimed that: "Eating just two carrots and two oranges a day will dramatically reduce heart disease. Fruit and vegetables contain anti-oxidants which stop the damaging effects of cholesterol. The Health Department recommends five serves a day to live longer."

The juxtaposition of this item with the science fiction tone of the blood washing story illustrates the pluralistic value of the news media: the unblinking ability to discuss the prevention of heart disease seconds apart framed in terms of two radically different metaphors and assumptions about the roles of biomedical treatment and lifestyle factors in prevention.

The most newsworthy story, the move to ban smoking in hotels and clubs (which featured on all television news bulletins on 16 March and reappeared throughout the sample week), also fitted into the low tech prevention narrative, but additionally incorporated elements of controversy based on apparent governmental authoritarianism and contempt for "the Australian way of life". In addition, it was a local story, combining state politics with health issues, two of the most newsworthy thematic categories for television news. A ban on smoking in enclosed public spaces is a decision that would attract great attention from health lobby groups who have campaigned for such a decision, and the tobacco and hotel industries who have strongly opposed it. The

ABC's news report framed the item almost wholly from the perspective of the latter, opening with the following statements:

Newsreader: Moves within State parliament for a blanket ban on smoking in all spaces except the home have sparked early protests in the hotel industry.
Reporter: It's as Australian as meat pies and kangaroos, but now the smoko at the local pub is under threat.
Male drinker: No, no, no. It's the last bastion.
Reporter: If Independent Peter McDonald has his way, indoor smoking will be outlawed everywhere except the private home or car. The fine, $5000.

The themes of hypocrisy on the part of politicians and the state's intrusion into everyday life were also taken up by the other three channels:

Channel 10: While the government has targeted the smoker, State Parliament remains one of the few public buildings where smoking is still permitted.
Channel 9: In another blow for smokers . . .
Channel 7 (Male smoker): Not in a pub or a club . . . 'cos . . . that's the only place you can really let your hair down, y'know?
Reporter: It's sacred?
Smoker: Yeah.

In this discourse, rather than frame the issue as a victory for health campaigners over the vested interests of the tobacco industry, or to describe the reaction from the two thirds majority of Australian non-smokers, the reporter and editors elected to frame smoking as a cherished national icon and a "last bastion" against the slippery slope of government health regulation. It was asserted inaccurately that individuals would face a $5000 fine, whereas this fine was in fact the potential maximum that would be imposed upon hotel or club owners, not smokers themselves.

Print media coverage of health and medicine

For the six months from January to June 1993, we gathered together press cuttings of health and medical items from leading

Table IV: Newspapers included in study of print media coverage of health and medicine in Sydney and the United Kingdom

Sydney, Jan–June 1993 (n = 4012)	Items	UK, Mar 1993 (n = 910)	Items
Daily Telegraph Mirror	1035	Independent[†]	124
Sydney Morning Herald	997	Telegraph[†]	108
Australian[†]	741	Daily Express[†]	91
Sunday Telegraph	286	The Times[†]	87
Sun Herald	278	Guardian	79
Woman's Day	154	Daily Mail[†]	69
New Idea	124	Mirror[†]	64
Ita	65	Sun[†]	52
Bulletin	61	Today	50
Time	61	Evening Standard	37
Women's Weekly	59	Other	37
Cosmopolitan	43	Daily Star	30
Cleo	41	Morning Star	25
WHO Weekly	37	Financial Times	21
Newsweek	16	Observer	17
Dolly	14	People	12
		News of the World	6

[†] Includes Sunday editions.

newspapers and women's and news magazines published in Sydney. We also obtained a full set of cuttings about health and medical issues from those supplied by commercial media monitoring services to the British Health Education Authority (covering the main British dailies) for the month of March 1993. Table IV shows our samples, and Table V lists the top 10 issues reported for both countries.

In the Sydney sample, reports of road injury and death, and of efforts to reduce the road toll, were a clear first. Injuries to people at work also rated highly, perhaps reflecting a media appetite for the "incident" hard news nature of traumatic injury. Three related issues concerning health care financing (political debate about the cost of health insurance, tales of run down hospital facilities and cuts to services, and a threatened strike by visiting medical specialists to public hospitals over pay cuts) also rated

Table V: *Top 10 issues reported in Sydney and British publications*

	Sydney, Jan–June 1993 ($n = 4012$)	Items		UK, Mar 1993 ($n = 910$)	Items
1.	Road injury	224	1.	AIDS and health care workers	148
2.	Medicine gone wrong: scientific and medical misconduct, negligence	217	2.	Health insurance	47
3.	Health insurance debate	161	3.	Sexual behaviour	46
4.	Hospital funding cuts	149	4.	Alcohol abuse and control	45
5.	Doctors' pay dispute	134	5.	Smoking cessation	43
6.	Passive smoking	119	6.	Tobacco and alcohol tax	35
7.	Transplant surgery, organ donations	82	7.	SIDS and SUDS	31
8.	Occupational injuries, health	80	8.	Scientific and medical misconduct, negligence	31
9.	AIDS education, campaigns, fund raising	79	9.	Condoms	30
10.	Life and death of Professor Fred Hollows	66	10.	Hospital funding cuts	28

SIDS = sudden infant death syndrome; SUDS = sudden unexplained death syndrome.

highly. These three stories generally contrasted the shame of alleged government neglect of public institutions of healing and nurturance with implications of the grasping venality of the highest paid echelons on the health care system, who were demanding even higher pay. The doctors, of course, often attempted (and succeeded) in appropriating the general subtext of government neglect in support of their own case.

The death of Professor Fred Hollows caused a concentration of reportage. Hollows had long fascinated the Australian media. He was the antithesis of almost every medical stereotype: a gnarled, pipe smoking, whiskey drinking, swearing, and bureaucrat bashing ophthalmologist, Hollows had for many years run a pioneering programme of treating eye disease in Aboriginal people in the dust and poverty of the outback. The juxtaposition of the intricacy and delicacy of his eye surgery work in restoring sight to some of the most underprivileged people on earth in some of the most testing physical environments (Eritrea, Nepal, Vietnam) complemented the authentic appeal of his personality. Anyone who might have blanched at his distance from the stereotype of the groomed, professional, and ultimately élite doctor, was forced to examine such prejudice against what he achieved. What *mattered* were the results of his work. Hollows was thus an icon to Australian values of contempt for élitism and formality, mistrust of bureaucrats, and of generosity towards those in need.

Of note was the greater frequency of health and medical stories run in women's magazines in Australia compared with those in news magazines such as *Time, Newsweek* and The *Bulletin*, while the tabloid *Daily Telegraph Mirror* published slightly more than the *Sydney Morning Herald*.

Table IV shows that, in the United Kingdom, quality broadsheet newspapers ran more health items than their tabloid rivals. Several of the leading issues shown in Table V, however, were reported most often in the tabloid papers. The "British disease" of sexual prurience and fascination for scandal, satirised so often in plays such as *No Sex Please, We're British!*, was plainly a factor in determining the make up of the top 10 health issues that were reported. One of the case studies following takes up the leading issue (the alleged threat of HIV infected doctors transmitting the virus to their patients). There was heavy reportage about a survey of sexual practices of British people, and an abundance of "outraged" reporting about schoolchildren's access to condoms.

The remainder of this chapter details four case studies of medical or public health issues making the news in Sydney and the United Kingdom. The two stories from the Australian press were included in the second leading topical category, "medicine gone wrong", whereas the two British case studies are from the first and fifth highest ranking categories.

Sydney stories

Creutzfeldt–Jakob disease

Creutzfeldt–Jakob Disease (CJD) is an extremely rare condition that has a latency period of up to 30 years, is untreatable, unscreenable, and can only be confirmed *post mortem*. It is transmitted by prions, virus-like particles that are carried in the blood.

Between January and June 1993, 18 press stories in Sydney newspapers and two lengthy feature articles in women's magazines were devoted to CJD, all related to the cases of four Australian women who had died of CJD between 1988 and 1991. The *Sydney Morning Herald* took a particular interest in the case, publishing most of the news stories.[14] The women affected by CJD had all been experiencing fertility difficulties and had been prescribed a new hormone treatment to stimulate ovulation. In the mid-1970s they were given free injections of human pituitary gonadotrophin (hPG), which had been extracted from the pituitary glands of corpses, as part of the National Human Pituitary Hormone Program, which ran between 1964 and 1985. The programme ceased operation in 1985 following the reports of two deaths in the United States from recipients of hPG.

Until the Australian news media began to cover these cases in late 1992, CJD had rarely received public attention. In January 1993, allegations by Dr Lynette Dumble and Dr Renate Klein, both medical researchers from Melbourne, were published in the *Medical Observer*, a medical magazine. The researchers claimed that recipients of blood donated by people who had received hPG treatment should be urgently traced, as the prions causing the disease could be transmitted via blood transfusions. The *Sydney Morning Herald* picked up the story, publishing articles with such headlines as: "WARNING OVER RARE BRAIN ILLNESS" (27 January 1993). The chairman of the National Blood Transfusion Committee responded by alleging that "there was 'no evidence' that CJD might be transmitted by blood transfusion" (*Sydney Morning Herald*, 27 January 1993). The following month, however, the Federal Government agreed to award the husbands of the dead women compensation, in a similar way in which the state admitted liability for people who had acquired HIV infection from transfused blood or blood products. Compensation was to be based on a formula including expenses for lost wages and hospital admissions. In May 1993, the Federal Minister for Health announced that an independent inquiry would be held into the use of hPG. In June, the first claims for damages by a person at risk from CJD following injection of hPG was filed. The woman sued the Commonwealth Government and Commonwealth Serum Laboratories for inducing psychological damage arising from stress, claiming that she had not been told of the risk of degenerative brain damage involved, that the drug had been extracted from dead bodies, or that the treatment was experimental. Three husbands of CJD victims also sued for damages, alleging negligence, claiming that the Commonwealth Serum Laboratories and the Department of Health knew, or ought to have known, about the potential risks of the treatment.

During this time, the rareness of the disease and its grisly origin—the hormone being derived from the brains of corpses —inspired such dramatic headlines as:

- LIVING WITH THE DEVIL (*Sydney Morning Herald*, 15 May 1993)
- FROM CORPSE BRAINS TO FEARS OF EPIDEMIC (*Australian*, 15 May 1993).

Other headlines focused on the growing (if still extremely small) death toll from CJD, collectively conveying an impression of a silently spreading disease:

- THIRD DEATH FOUND FROM HORMONE TREATMENT (*Sydney Morning Herald*, 30 January 1993)
- FOURTH DEATH FROM FERTILITY PROGRAM (*Daily Telegraph Mirror*, 1 May 1993)
- WOMAN CONFIRMED AS FOURTH CJD VICTIM (*Sydney Morning Herald*, 1 May 1993)

- NEW DEATH TRIGGERS HORMONE INQUIRY (*Sydney Morning Herald*, 12 May 1993)
- HUNDREDS MORE IN HORMONE TRIAL SCARE (*Sydney Morning Herald*, 15 May 1993),

as did such sentences as: "A stealthy, incurable killer is taking a tragic toll of Australian women. Worse may be in store: researchers fear cases of medically acquired Creutzfeldt–Jakob disease, an insidious condition that slowly and irreversibly destroys the brain, may be revealing a hidden epidemic" (*Australian*, 15 May 1993).

The disease also gave the press an opportunity to dramatise and personalise the stories of its victims. For example, in a three page article published in the women's magazine *New Idea* (5 June 1993), people affected by CJD were interviewed. The article, headed "THE SILENT KILLER" centred around the fear and anxiety generated by not knowing if one's body was harbouring a potentially fatal disease. The lead sentence noted, "Isabelle lives with the fear that she will die an excruciating death from the rare but fatal brain disorder, Creutzfeldt–Jakob disease, or CJD . . . 'It's as if you are always preparing for death,' says Isabelle, 40."

The article emphasised the lack of knowledge about the potential risks involved experienced by recipients: "If I had known I never would have done it, Isabelle says . . . Noel, 50, alleges that he and [his wife] Jenny were never warned of health risks involved with using the fertility hormone. 'If you've waited 10 years to have children, you'll put your faith in anything,' he says."

The article went on to allege that the two medical scientists who had brought CJD to light had received threats following their revelations: " 'It is the most unethical coverup,' says Dr Dumble . . . 'The moral responsibility should come first—to admit that a treatment has gone diabolically wrong.' . . . The doctors say they have stuck with the issue 'to help give those who've been treated with these hormones the respect and specific care they deserve. Science without social conscience is a deadly enemy' [they said]."

Another long article published in the June 1993 issue of *Ita* magazine, a publication aimed at middle aged women, asserted,

"Women who took part in a government-sponsored hormone programme that is being blamed for three deaths are living on a razor's edge because of a bureaucratic wall of silence" and interviewed a woman who had received hPG, quoting her as saying, "When I tried to obtain information from the Commonwealth Department of Health, I came across a wall of silence that makes me wonder whether they are trying hard to cover something up." Articles in the *Sydney Morning Herald* also centred around the issue of state responsibility, as in this lead sentence: "The husbands of two women who were the first to die from a rare brain disease linked to a human hormone treatment for infertility have called for a high-level inquiry into what they claim may be Australia's worst medical disaster" (11 February 1993).

That newspaper's headlines emphasised the search for blame and retribution:

- COMPO CALL OVER HORMONE DEATHS (4 February 1993)
- WIDOWERS SEEK INQUIRY INTO DONOR BRAIN DISEASE (11 February 1993)
- THE SEARCH FOR BLAME (24 February 1993)
- NEW CALL FOR CJD DEATHS INQUIRY (8 March 1993).

This advocacy case was led by two feminist medical researchers and three husbands of women who had contracted CJD. Even though very few people were known to be affected by the disease, the issue won attention because of the following factors.

- Novelty: the disease was previously unheard of and extremely rare.
- Seriousness: the disease caused degeneration of the most valorised organ of the body, the brain, leading to death, and struck young people down before their time.
- Potential for an inexorably growing epidemic: it was alleged that thousands of Australians, who may have received infected blood from blood transfusions or organ transplants, could have CJD lying hidden in their bodies.
- The bizarre: hPG had been extracted from dead bodies.
- The ideology of motherhood: the disease had killed only women thus far, all of whom were relatively young and had

used hPG in the attempt to conceive, and some of whom had left young families behind.

- The health of infants was implicated: there were also suggestions made that the disease could be passed from mother to fetus *in utero*.
- Conflict and blame: the search for those organisations or individuals responsible for the women's deaths.
- Cover-up and corruption: allegations were made of the government attempting to evade its responsibility and threats made against the medical researchers who were attempting to draw attention to the issue.

Because of these newsworthy properties, the husbands of women who had died from CJD were able to attract press attention to their calls for an inquiry into the reasons why there was no tight control over who received the hormones and considerable support for their claim for compensation. Their efforts were vastly aided by the coverage given to the issue by the *Sydney Morning Herald*, a prestigious newspaper with a history of investigative journalism uncovering corruption and medical negligence, which took up the cause of the victims of CJD and their families and called valuable attention to the alleged neglect of the Department of Health on their behalf.

Breast implants

The issue of the health side effects of silicone gel breast implants has attracted a high level of news media over the past three years. In early 1993 it was reported that over 200 Australian women sought to sue the American manufacturers of the implants, Dow Corning Corporation, in a class action to add to the thousands of American women seeking compensation through their country's courts. The side effects for women who had received silicone gel implants mentioned in news reports included scleroderma (thickening and hardening of tissue), lupus erythematosus (an autoimmune condition), chronic fatigue syndrome, pain, psychological distress, immune system irregularities, "poisoning" of the body, "crippling fatigue", and the need for further invasive surgery. By early 1993 it was emerging that it was not only the health of women who had received faulty implants that was placed in jeopardy, but also perhaps that of their children. It was reported that tests had found unusually high silicone levels in the blood of infants breast fed by their mothers who had had implants. One woman was quoted as saying, "I want to know if I have given my children a life sentence. Are they going to live, and for how long?" (*Sydney Morning Herald*, 24 June 1993) and headlines such as "HIGH SILICONE IN BABY'S BLOOD" (*Daily Telegraph Mirror*, 23 June 1993) and "NEW FEARS FOR IMPLANT MOTHERS" (*Sydney Morning Herald*, 24 June 1993) appeared.

In the articles on breast implants that appeared in the newspapers and magazines surveyed, it is notable the discursive strategies employed that reproduced a number of stereotypes concerning femininity. For example, the emphasis in several stories was on women's emotions—their difficulty in coping with their anxiety, their anger, their depression, their fear for their own and their children's health. Reports referred to the "worry", "guilt" and "psychological damage" experienced by women who had received implants, as in the following extracts:

Hundreds of confused and angry women bombarded the Women's Implant Information Network yesterday . . . "We've had women ringing and ringing, confused and in tears." (*Daily Telegraph Mirror*, 13 April 1993)

When she heard the results of the silicon test on her son she felt "just sick in the stomach and you feel a real sense of guilt, I guess. I just went into a pretty depressed state." (*Sydney Morning Herald*, 24 June 1993)

Headlines also focused on the emotional response of women "victims":

● MORE WORRY FOR BREAST IMPLANT VICTIMS (*Sun Telegraph*, 17 January 1993)
● WOMEN IN UPROAR OVER $1BN CLAIM (*Daily Telegraph Mirror*, 13 April 1993)
● BREAST IMPLANT PAYOUT STIRS AUST WOMEN (*Sydney Morning Herald*, 17 April 1993).

The femininity of the women involved was emphasised, especially in magazine articles: "Fran Bates has a soft, low voice . . ." (*Who Weekly*, 10 May 1993), as was their status as passive victims: "the implants may have robbed her of her life"

(*Who Weekly*, 10 May 1993). In other women's magazine articles, famous women's cases were detailed—"Actor Jessica Lange has had her silicone breast boosters secretly removed and replaced with safer, smaller saline implants to avoid poisonous gel leaking into her body" (*New Idea*, 19 June 1993)—yet juxtaposed with descriptions of other plastic surgery procedures that "made the stars smile" and the use of before and after photographs to show the results that "speak for themselves"—Faye Dunaway's facelift, Jane Fonda's "breast job" and facelift, and Lisa Hartman's "nose job". Such stories implied that cosmetic surgery itself was not problematic, only that surgery that is poorly performed. News reports also implied this: "Women are being denied the chance to have silicon-free breast enlargements because doctors are unaware of or misinformed about the procedure, plastic surgeons said yesterday" (*Daily Telegraph Mirror*, 12 May 1993).

Indeed, one article published in the *Sydney Morning Herald* (12 May 1993) with the headline, "NEW BREAST HAS TUMMY TUCK BONUS", reporting a new method of breast reconstruction for women who have had a mastectomy involving the removal and use of abdominal tissue, served to trivialise the issue. A plastic surgeon was quoted as saying: "We take a little muscle from just below the pubic area and as most Western women have extra fat in the abdominal area—particularly after having babies—they get a tummy tuck as well."

Thus, although the hazardous side effects of silicone gel implants were emphasised in press accounts, there was very little challenge to the underlying belief that cosmetic surgery is appropriate to make women feel better about themselves.

Juxtaposed with the representation of individual women as passive and irrationally emotional victims was a contradictory portrayal of women collectively as active agents, forming together in a consumer group to challenge a large, US based corporation and seek legal redress for their plight—for example, although the *Who Weekly* article's lead sentence described women as "shattered that breast implants could be poisoning them" it went on to say that "Australian women want answers." The *Daily Telegraph Mirror* (13 April 1993), even while describing women as in "anguish", "confused", "in tears" and "poisoned" with silicone, also described them as "fighting a protracted battle" with Dow Corning and quoted one woman as saying,

"We want help, not false promises." It was reported that affected women had established a Women's Implant Information Network to draw attention to their problem and provide support for others. Even though when Dow Corning responded by offering to pay for women to have their implants removed in private hospitals (although still not admitting legal liability of any kind), a series of headlines in Sydney newspapers represented the corporation as "helping" women and responding to their claims:

- BREAST IMPLANT MAKER OFFERS REMOVAL HELP (*Sydney Morning Herald*, 12 January 1993)
- DOW TO PAY FOR IMPLANT FAILURES (*The Australian*, 12 January 1993)
- IMPLANT FIRM OFFERS HELP (*Daily Telegraph Mirror*, 12 January 1993)
- SILICONE BREAST IMPLANT OFFER (*Sydney Morning Herald*, 13 January 1993).

Most articles went on to detail the Information Network's cynical response to the company's offer. The *Sun Telegraph* (17 January 1993) quoted the director of the Network, Fran Bates, as being "sceptical about the extent of [Dow Corning's] assistance and says it is too late for many", while the *Sydney Morning Herald* (13 January 1993) noted that "The Women's Implant Information Network demanded yesterday to know if Dow Corning Australia planned to match the US offer—$1200 to each woman—or offer more money."

The newsworthy properties of the story included the following.

- The pain of achieving feminine beauty—the wages of vanity.
- The issue concerned both the enhancement and the deformation of breasts, an important bodily site of femininity and sexuality.
- Famous women suffering from the side effects of implants.
- Medical negligence—plastic surgeons caring more about income than about their patients' health.
- Medical control over women's bodies.
- The imputed threat to small infants' health status via their mother's implants.

- Young mothers fearing for their ability to care for their children properly because of the disabling side effects of their alleged silicone "poisoning".
- The fear associated with having "foreign" matter inside one's body, causing hidden damage by silently leaking into bodily tissues and the blood stream.
- The scandal involved with a large multinational corporation allegedly refusing to take responsibility for the health side effects of its products.
- The conflict engendered by the efforts of a small group of "ordinary" Australian women attempting to challenge big business.

The breast implant story thus provided an example of an advocacy issue receiving news attention largely through the personalisation of the plight of individual women and the use of subtexts emerging from stereotypical representations of "femininity" and "motherhood". Because women had taken the step of forming an advocacy group—the Women's Implant Information Network—which gave them a collective "voice" that could respond to Dow Corning's actions and provide quotes for journalists, there was the opportunity to use the media to counteract the "passive victim" portrayal and work towards pressuring the corporation and the state to act on the matter.

British stories

Doctors with HIV/AIDS

In terms of quantity of news stories generated, the top issue in the British press sampled in the month of March was that involving the revelation that a number of doctors in England and Wales had continued to practise medicine while knowing they were infected with HIV, including a gynaecologist and paediatrician.

These announcements raised related issues of the need to test health care workers for HIV and prompted the announcement by the British Health Secretary, Virginia Bottomley, that there would be an urgent review of guidelines relating to British health authorities' handling of such cases. It is interesting that this issue was so newsworthy that the Australian news media also picked up on it, with one current affairs programme devoting a lengthy segment to discussing the story and its relevance for Australians (see the earlier discussion in this chapter).

Central to the newsworthiness of this story was the notion of doctors as threats of HIV transmission to their patients. Opinion pieces argued that "I certainly wouldn't want any surgeon of mine to be suffering from AIDS" (*Daily Mail*, 10 March 1993) and the *Daily Express* (10 March 1993) asserted:

[The HIV-positive gynaecologist] did hysterectomies and delivered babies, dealing with women at their most trusting and vulnerable. When there is patients' blood, the cut finger of an HIV-positive doctor can end a life. Or, in the labour ward, two lives. We should test the medical men and women who operate on us for HIV.

The association of members of the medical profession with "deviant" behaviour such as homosexuality was also a source of newsworthiness; for example, the *Sun*'s headline trumpeted "SEX SHAME OF SURGEON: HE HAD CONVICTIONS FOR CHATTING UP MEN" (11 March 1993). Not surprisingly, the news apparently created panic and anxiety among some of the patients who had been treated by the doctors in question. Women were said to have "flooded a hospital helpline" after photographs of one doctor were published in newspapers (*Evening Standard*, 9 March 1993). The *Daily Mirror*'s headline read "4,000 WOMEN IN FEAR JAM AIDS DOC PHONES" (8 March 1993), while articles that same day in the *Sun*, *Today* and *Daily Express* newspapers featured stories with the headlines "MUMS' FURY AT AIDS DOCTOR COVER UP", "THOUSANDS OF MOTHERS DEMAND: GIVE US AIDS TESTS" and "MOTHERS IN PANIC ON AIDS SURGEON" respectively. The *Sunday Mail* chose to personalise the story by featuring a woman who had attended one of the doctor's surgeries:

I am a wife and mother of two beautiful children. Last week my life was turned upside down. Why? Because I believed that a doctor I trusted had put me at risk from a life-threatening disease . . . I kept asking myself: Why should my husband and I be put at risk, however small, by the medical profession we rely on to keep us healthy?

As did the *Sun* (9 March 1993): "Mum Kathleen Smith, waiting for the result of her AIDS test, sobbed: 'I have been crying since my husband told me about this. I knew straight away he had done my op[eration]. He could have known about this for years.'"

Later that month there were accompanying stories fuelling further discussion of the issue, including reports that a general practitioner who worked in a Lancashire hospital casualty department had died of AIDS related illnesses, a London dentist had continued to work after his HIV positive status became known, and an eminent paediatrician who had died two years previously had been HIV positive. Headlines noted:

- CASUALTY DOC DIES OF AIDS (*News of the World*, 14 March 1993)
- ANOTHER DOCTOR DIES OF AIDS (*Sunday Express*, 14 March 1993)
- I WORKED ON DESPITE HIV, SAYS DENTIST (*Evening Standard*, 12 March 1993)
- HIV DENTIST TELLS: WHY I WORKED ON (*Daily Express*, 13 March 1993)
- GAY DENTIST KEPT HIV SECRET FOR 6 MONTHS (*Today*, 13 March 1993)
- CHILD DOCTOR DIED OF AIDS (*Today*, 17 March 1993)
- ANOTHER DOCTOR IN HIV DEATH (*Daily Telegraph*, 17 March 1993)
- TOP KID'S DOC DIED OF AIDS (*Daily Mirror*, 17 March 1993)
- CHILD ABUSE EXPERT'S DEATH LINKED TO AIDS (*Daily Mail*, 17 March 1993).

Features and opinion pieces accused the medical profession and other health care workers of hypocrisy, evasion, closed ranks, and lack of consideration for their patients' wellbeing. This approach was especially prominent in the tabloid newspapers. For example, the *Daily Mirror* (17 March 1993) commented, "Covering up, whatever the potential embarrassment, doesn't work; looks shifty, and in the case of the AIDS-infected doctors, has contributed hugely to the current panic and confusion", while the *Daily Express*'s headline claimed that "MEDICS SHOULD LIFT THE MASK" (17 March 1993) and went on to argue that "The medical profession has policed itself and pleased itself for too long. It's time some public accountability was injected."

The chief fear, as expressed in these accounts, was that an HIV positive doctor might bleed into an open wound while operating, perhaps after suffering a needle stick injury or small cut during surgery. Subsequently several articles called for compulsory HIV antibody testing of doctors and other health workers.

What these arguments failed to acknowledge is that the procedures taken by medical practitioners and other health care workers to minimise spreading infection of any contagious agent, including the wearing of surgical gloves and masks, also prevents the likelihood of HIV transmission via such a route. They also neglected the fact that there had been no documented case in Western countries of a doctor transmitting HIV to a patient, that the vast majority of doctor–patient interactions does not involve contact with blood (including most routine gynaecological examinations), that testing of health care workers would have to take place regularly and would therefore be exorbitantly expensive, and that HIV infection usually does not show up on HIV antibody tests in the first three months anyway. Very few newspapers discussed such details; one of the few articles to do so was published in the *Guardian* (12 March 1993), which noted, "Health care workers face greater risk of HIV infection in their work than patients coming into contact with doctors, nurses or midwives" and, "There are no documented instances of a doctor, midwife or nurse transmitting HIV to a patient." An opinion piece in the *Observer* (14 March 1993) also cautioned against knee-jerk panic and punitive responses, arguing: "No British doctor has ever infected a patient. So why should they be tested?", while *The Times* (16 March 1993) also supported the medical profession, arguing: "The doctor who listens to and taps your chest, peers down your throat and looks into your ears or who takes your smear or feels your prostate will never give you anything more sinister than a cold or 'flu."

Members of the health services bureaucracy were also taken to task in the British newspapers for their alleged attempts to "cover up" their knowledge of the doctors' HIV positive status. Again the tabloids were in the forefront of criticism—for example, an article published in the *Sun* (15 March 1993) was headed "SCANDAL OF AIDS DOC COVER-UP" and began: "A doctor dying of AIDS hid his disease from hospital bosses—and his partners helped in the cover-up, it was revealed yesterday. The man worked in a big city practice with other GPs who knew of his condition and put up a wall of silence."

The *Daily Star* (18 March 1993) said:

Having had it drummed into us that sex without a condom is like jumping out of a plane without a parachute, we now find you don't have to have sex at all to catch AIDS. If you want to live dangerously, go to hospital—as dozens of doctors now have the virus. And to make matters worse, their bloody employers have the cheek to try and hide it from us.

Other articles were headlined:

- FURY AT AIDS COVER-UP (*Today*, 11 March 1993)
- DOCTOR'S DEATH FROM AIDS KEPT SECRET FOR FIVE MONTHS (*The Guardian*, 11 March 1993)
- AIDS DOCTOR SECRECY ROW (*Daily Mail*, 15 March 1993)
- DOCTOR NO. 3 KEPT DEADLY AIDS SECRET (*Daily Star*, 15 March 1993)
- AIDS COVER-UP BY DOCTORS (*Daily Express*, 15 March 1993)
- SILENCE OVER AIDS GP (*Daily Telegraph*, 15 March 1993)
- GP KEPT ILLNESS SECRET FROM HOSPITAL CHIEFS (*Today*, 15 March 1993)
- AIDS DOCTOR NAMED AS ANGRY PATIENTS HIT OUT (*Daily Express*, 16 March 1993)
- STOP DOCTORING THE TRUTH: TELL US WHO HAS AIDS (*Daily Star*, 18 March 1993)

Similar statements were made expressing concern about the actions engaged in by the health authority and other doctors involved. The use of the words "scandal", "fury", "row" and "angry" in the headlines and main texts are overtly emotive and imply conflict, while the recurring use of the words "cover-up", "secrecy", "secret" and "silence" fuelled the "conspiracy" theory, casting the medical profession and British health authorities not only as incompetent but also as deceitful.

This issue was newsworthy because it incorporated the following.

- Fears about contagion and casual contact with respect to HIV/AIDS—sources of concern ever since the first emergence of the epidemic—were raised again by the threat of this "new" potential route of transmission.
- The revelations of "cover-ups" cast doubt on the integrity of the medical profession and the health services bureaucracy.
- The issue raised concerns of imputed risk to pregnant women/mothers and small children because a gynaecologist and paediatrician were involved.

- The numbers of patients involved: thousands of people who had been treated over the years by the doctors appeared to panic and fear for their lives once they were aware of the revelations of the doctors' seropositivity.
- Anxiety was created around a relationship—the doctor–patient relationship—which relies upon trust and faith to function.
- The issue was conflictive, implying a schism between doctors/authorities (as villains) and patients (as victims).
- The issue allowed the tabloid press in particular to express anti-authoritarian sentiments.

Smoking cessation

Britain's National No Smoking Day fell during the study period (on 10 March 1993) and there were a large number of news stories generated around this event and related issues of smoking cessation. The event was launched by Virginia Bottomley, who authoritatively announced, "My job is to say to everybody, and above all to parents, 'Quit it'." In response, however, a number of Conservative backbenchers tabled a motion that criticised state efforts to control smoking and "the sweeping nanny state persecution of smoking minorities" and defiantly lit their pipes at a special lunch held for smokers in Parliament. As a result, Bottomley was cast in the role of "Nanny", and represented in most articles as a strict, authoritarian "goody-goody". The *Daily Express* (11 March 1993), for example, published a photograph of her with the somewhat familiar headline, "GOLDEN VIRGINIA" and spoke of her "best headmistressy tones" and the way she had "nagged" her husband into giving up smoking "as an example to their three children." The *Daily Star*'s headline announced that "FUMING MPS BLAST 'NANNY' GINNY OVER NO SMOKING DAY" and quoted Lord Mason, a former Labour Cabinet minister as saying, "It is a pity that intolerant elements in our society are seeking to impose their anti-smoking opinions on our democratic society." That same day, newspapers also reported that BAT, a major multinational tobacco company, had announced record profits from sale of their cigarettes, publishing photographs of executives from that company smiling gleefully.

Another common representation was that of smokers as social

87

outcasts and recalcitrants. The *Independent* (11 March 1993), for example, published photographs of three furtive-looking male smokers caught in the act, describing them as "Three men ignoring the high moral ground on National No Smoking Day." An article in *The Times* (11 March 1993) described the "deviant" status of smokers forced to hide their habit, but also provided quotes from defiant smokers determined to ignore the warnings of public health officials:

Huddled on street corners yesterday were bands of undercover smokers, hounded out of the many offices and institutions in the City of London where smoking has been banned . . . "I've smoked for almost 40 years and no one but me is going to decide when I quit," said Leonard Dexter, a 25-a-day man.

Celebrities and prominent people were particularly called to task for their insistence on smoking, perhaps because of their potential to act as influential "role models", especially for children. Bill Wyman, ex-member of the Rolling Stones, was caught on camera smoking a cigarette before playing at a charity concert, held, ironically enough, to raise funds for the British Lung Foundation. Unflattering photographs of the "ageing rocker" illustrated stories published in the tabloids on 13 March 1993 with headlines such as "FAGGED OUT BILL'S ASH CASH" (*Daily Mirror*), "PUFFING BILLY LIGHTS UP A CHARITY BALL" (*Today*) and "STRIKE A LIGHT! IT'S BILL AT A LUNG CANCER CHARITY NIGHT" (*Sun*). A columnist in the *Daily Express* (12 March 1993) discussed Home Secretary Kenneth Clarke's predilection for smoking cigars in Parliament in disapproving and comical terms, emphasised by a photograph of Clarke blowing smoke with the caption, "There he blows: Kenneth with his cigar" and asserting, "Being adjacent during the working day to a constantly smouldering cigarillo or whatever, is about as conducive to health, happiness and fragrantly smelling hair as being stationed closely behind an elderly, curry-eating, Afghan mountain goat with terminal gastroenteritis."

The *Sun* (10 March 1993) castigated Princess Margaret for her smoking habit, publishing a photograph of her looking wan, drawn, and worried (but *sans* cigarette) with the accusing headline "HOW MANY DID YOU HAVE TODAY?" The article went on to use outrageous puns to censure the Princess for her habit:

Princess Margaret is just back from a Caribbean holiday. Butt [sic] who'd have known from her fagged-out look last night? The 62-year-old royal was clearly a little puffy . . . as though she may be still on the ciggies despite her recent health scare . . . her docs may be wondering if she's really given up!

The *Sun* had earlier that month also published an article on the death of Lord Ridley, an ex-member of Margaret Thatcher's cabinet, with the headline: "A GREAT ENGLISHMAN: MAGGIE'S GRIEF AS 80 CIGS A DAY KILL HER FRIEND RIDLEY" (6 March 1993). The photograph published with the article showed Ridley with a cigarette hanging out of his mouth and the caption, "Lord Ridley . . . died of lung cancer at the age of 64." It was noted, "He even puffed during Cabinet [and] smoked four packs of Silk Cut a day." That same newspaper referred back to Ridley's death in a short opinion piece on No Smoking Day which asserted:

I hope any of you still puffing on the fags saw the last appearance Nicholas Ridley made in the House of Lords, shown on the news the day he died. An 80-a-day man, his agonised rasping for breath would surely have made you draw your breath in sharply too.

The Times editorial on Ridley's death was headlined "A DEADLY HABIT" and went on to comment, "Lord Ridley died as he lived, relishing his politics and his cigarettes to the very end."

More ordinary mortals continued to be condemned for their smoking activities in a series of articles that reported research findings casting smokers as self deluding, a danger to others, bad parents, or even sexually incompetent. The *Daily Express*, for example, published an article headlined "MUMS WHO SMOKE RATHER THAN SMACK" about women who "ignore health risks to their families because they wrongly think cigarettes make them calmer" (8 March 1993) and also an article called "DEADLY LEGACY OF THE FATHERS WHO SMOKE" (6 March 1993), which went on to say that men could be harming their children and even their grandchildren by smoking, because of birth defects, genetic defects, cancer, or early death. *Today* (10 March 1993) published an article about children who begged their parents to give up smoking:

89

PLEASE GIVE UP SMOKING, MUM

A girl of five summed up the agony of children who fear their parents could smoke themselves into an early grave. Hannah Crisp marked today's No Smoking Day with the touching plea: "I want my mum to stop smoking because she will die and she is only 34."

On 25 March several newspapers reported the assertions of the British Agencies for Adoption and Fostering that babies should not be placed in households with smokers, using headlines such as "SMOKERS CAN'T ADOPT" (*Daily Mail*) and "SMOKING 'SHOULD BE A BAR TO ADOPTION'" (*Daily Telegraph*). The *Daily Star* reported on men who were "TOO FAGGED FOR NOOKIE" (13 March 1993), asserting, "Men who smoke risk being a big FLOP in bed" and the *Daily Mirror* published a short item headlined "FAT CHANCE" which noted, "Fatties, smokers and boasters are the least likely people to find a bedmate, an American sex survey has revealed" (5 March 1993).

In addition to these articles representing smokers highly punitively (without any consideration of the commercial and socioeconomic environment in which smokers are persuaded to take up and maintain the habit) several articles published around No Smoking Day gave some useful advice for people wanting to give up. The *Independent* (8 March 1993) and *The Times* (9 March 1993) both published feature articles on the difficulties of giving up smoking, acknowledging the complex reasons why people find it hard to give up permanently, while others such as the *Daily Express* (9 March 1993), *Daily Mirror* (10 March 1993) and *Daily Mail* (9 March 1993) provided tips for ways of stopping smoking, giving personalised stories of smokers who had successfully quit using different methods.

To sum up, the newsworthy aspects of this issue included:

- Smokers as "deviants"—the new social outcasts.
- No Smoking Day, which provided a "hook" for articles about smoking both before, during and after it fell.
- Famous or prominent people being called to task for indulging in the habit.
- The conflict of the "nanny state" argument, revolving around people's rights to smoke if they so desire, and the "health promotion" argument, which focused on the utilitarian benefits if as many people as possible desist from smoking.

- Related to the above point but more specifically, the clash of opinions between politicians—Health Minister Virginia Bottomley as authoritarian, and anti-authoritarian responses to No Smoking Day on the part of her fellow Conservatives.
- The opportunity for newspapers to perform a social service by providing information and hints about giving up smoking.

Discussion

The case studies examined in this chapter provide important pointers for those involved in public health advocacy, especially with regard to the principles of newsworthiness. The frames placed around health and medical issues that we uncovered in our case studies have significant implications for news audiences' and readers' construction of lay understandings about such issues. News stories dealing with issues around life and death matters, or even events or developments relating to lifestyle choices, often presenting confusing and conflicting information. Television news is believed by many people to be the most credible of all news sources. Yet the average length of screen time of the news stories we surveyed was only 67 seconds. Credibility then, would seem to have little to do with comprehensiveness but more to do with the coalescence of visually striking images, dramatic headlines, and the casting of stories within a limited number of frames and discourses, which better allow audiences to "make sense" rapidly of often technically and ethically complex health or medical topics. Although we would not argue that audiences absorb such messages passively, uncritically, or uniformly, as we noted in the previous chapter, the discursive ways in which media texts are structured and the language and images chosen during production, work to set up a hierarchy of discourses and persuade audiences to accept the producers' intended meaning.

As the Sydney television study showed, the bizarre, the moral warning, the discrediting of high status individuals, the medico-scientific breakthrough and the contrasting low tech reaffirmation of folk remedies or preventive measures provided the narratives around which almost all of the news stories in this sample were constructed. It is notable, however, that apart from

91

the one story on banning smoking in pubs and clubs, medical breakthroughs and bizarre bodies were given more attention than preventive items. This can be explained not only because of the "miraculous" nature of medical breakthroughs and the prurient voyeurism inspired by the bizarre, but also by the fact that preventive stories offer little in the way of arresting visual images. Viewers cannot "see" a healthy diet working to prevent against heart disease in the same way as they can witness heart surgery being performed by the high priests of medicine, clustered around an operating table with the very organ pulsing in their bloodied hands.

As a vehicle for one-way communication, television allows its audiences to make vicarious observations of intriguing, ordinarily inaccessible situations where their actual physical presence might result in consequences they would prefer to avoid. The codes of interpersonal conduct which apply in face to face encounters can be suspended when one is viewing others through a television screen. There are no risks involved, for example, in gazing intently at others' on-screen sexual behaviour, eavesdropping on others' filmed conversations or in expressing reactions that would normally be suppressed through concern for the response or feelings of those involved. In a society obsessed with the body—its attractiveness, sexual exploits, shape, state of health—and preoccupied with notions of physical risk and self discipline, the health and medical fields offer a wealth of opportunities for people to participate vicariously in many such taboo situations: one can stare or gawp unconstrainedly at the bodily misfortunes of others, learn of the private medical problems of strangers, and bear witness to medical procedures normally shrouded in medical privacy. Also worthy of note is television's tendency to cast heroes, villains, and victims in health and medical stories, both to trivialise some illnesses and magnify the importance of others in the quest for visually striking images, and to make moral judgements about ill people (especially those with HIV infection), thus promoting either sentimental sympathy or fatuous antipathy for their plight.

The newspaper studies also demonstrated several key points for public health advocates. One of these, particularly exemplified by the British press news stories, was that different types of newspapers report the same issues from different perspectives, obviously with their own readership in mind. The British tabloids, for example, were far more condemning of the medical profession over the issue of HIV positive doctors and health care workers than were the broadsheets, and their headlines in particular sought to inspire panic and cast doctors as villains. In general they were more willing to take an anti-authoritarian stance than were the broadsheets. The length of news stories is also closely related to the type of publication in which they appear. Magazine articles are frequently several pages long, while feature articles in "quality" broadsheets are usually in smaller print, less reliant on photographs, often more detailed and more considered of the issues involved, particularly if they are controversial, and tend to include many more news actors and news sources than those on the same topic in the popular tabloids. It is important for advocates to bear in mind the different types of stories that tend to receive attention in the different genres of newspapers when designing their campaigns, and to monitor which publications are likely to publish more health and medical stories than others, in order to be aware of the most receptive avenues for attempts to make the news.

The recurring narratives that emerged in the studies of press reports were those related to deviance, conspiracy, medical negligence, the insidious spread of disease, stereotypes of femininity and motherhood, the threat to young children, the search for blame, bureaucratic incompetence and anti-authoritarianism (particularly on the part of the British tabloid press). In most cases, the "patient" or "ordinary person" was set up in opposition to the "medical profession" or "bureaucrat", with emphasis on the rights of the former to access information or receive compensation for wrongs. Under such a framing, lay people were able to draw attention to their plight or concern, but often at the expense of the unidimensional stereotyping of members of the medical profession or health authorities as villains. Health advocates need to be wary of perpetuating this binary opposition because, although it meets the purposes of newsworthiness well, it also serves to cast blame unfairly, set up an antagonistic and unproductive relationship between "them" and "us" and creates individual scapegoats (the case of the medical practitioners with HIV/AIDS being a salutary case in point).

Although media advocacy is about directing the spotlight towards the causes of ill health that are traditionally obscured from public view, advocates need to work with, rather than against, the medical profession and health services bureaucracy, and should save their most virulent scapegoating strategies for commercial interests, for example, the tobacco and other drug industries, which continue to produce commodities that lead to ill health in the name of maximising profits. Likewise, it is counter-productive and ethically dubious to "victim blame" both ordinary and prominent individuals for their lifestyle habits (for example, the British tabloids' relentless hounding of Princess Margaret, Lord Ridley and Bill Wyman). Not only will such hounding engender ill will on the part of many members of the public and the individuals themselves, but the major concern of public health advocates should be emphasising the socioeconomic structural and institutional causes of ill health rather than the victimisation of individuals.

To conclude, it is clear that the visual impact of an event or issue and its scope for personalisation, or centring the story around an individual, in concert with the potential to slot the event into one or more existing newsworthy themes or narratives, is vital to its chances of making the news. Advocates interested in reframing health issues and attracting the attention and awareness of the public and policy makers need to be cognisant of these properties of news and be able to work within them. However, they must also be alert to ethical issues, including the dangers of victim blaming and scapegoating, and the risk of inciting media attention to an issue and then losing control over the way in which it is subsequently framed. Trivialising or oversimplification of the issue may ultimately prove counterproductive—not all news *is* good news.

References

1 Grundy B. Where is the news? A content analysis of a week's television news in Australia. In: Edgar P, editor. *The news in focus. The journalism of exception.* Melbourne: Macmillan, 1980.
2 Henningham J. *Looking at television news.* Melbourne: Longman Cheshire, 1988.

3 Brown WT. Progeria: a human-disease model of accelerated aging. *Am J Clin Nutr* 1992; 55 (6 suppl): 1222–4S.
4 Wang SM, Nishigori CK, Zhang JM, Takebe H. Reduced DNA-repair capacity in cells originating from a progeria patient. *Mutat Res* 1990; **237**: 253–7.
5 Hearst N, Hulley SB. Preventing the heterosexual spread of AIDS. *JAMA* 1988; **259**: 2428.

4: Case studies in public health media advocacy

SIMON CHAPMAN

In this chapter, I present two detailed case studies in media advocacy, both from New South Wales, Australia. They illustrate the ways in which proponents and opponents of two public health policies sought to advance their respective causes. The first describes a protracted public battle involving people concerned to prevent childhood drownings in domestic swimming pools through the compulsory installation of fences that would prevent unsupervised access by infants to backyard pools. Their opponents were a lobby group of pool owners who, concerned about the aesthetics of their garden landscaping, vigorously resisted the introduction of a law that would require all domestic swimming pools to be fenced. The second concerns a concerted attempt by the tobacco industry in the state to defeat a legislative proposal to ban all remaining forms of tobacco advertising and sponsorship.

Case study 1: garden aesthetics versus children's lives: media advocacy for the prevention of childhood drowning

This is an emotional issue, but experts on the prevention of avoidable childhood deaths are the ones to whom we should really pay attention.[1] (Then Premier of NSW, Nick Greiner supporting the requirement that all domestic pools have isolation fencing, June 1990.)

You can use facts to support any point of view on this issue, from saying it is entirely a parental responsibility to suggesting that every pool ought to have isolation fencing.[2] (Nick Greiner after rejecting the advice of experts on the prevention of avoidable childhood deaths and supporting the abolition of the requirement for isolation fencing, May 1992.)

On 2 July 1992, the New South Wales (NSW) Parliament passed the Swimming Pools Act (1992), replacing the Swimming Pool Fencing Act (1990). The principal provision of the new Act was to remove the requirement for all existing private pools to have isolation fencing erected by 1 August 1992. This action followed a two year campaign by the Pool Fencing Action Group (PFAG), a lobby group of pool owners opposed to isolation fencing, and negated more than 15 years of pro-fence advocacy work by paediatricians and public health workers, designed to reduce the incidence of child drowning.

This case study is an analysis of the ways in which the proponents and opponents of this requirement attempted to frame their positions via the media in their efforts to capture the dominant symbols of debate that would determine its public reception and set the agenda for its political fate. We conclude with an analysis of the rejection of the isolation fencing requirement and the implications arising for future public health advocacy efforts in this area.

Background

Drowning is the leading cause of death among one to four year olds in Australia.[3] Other water oriented societies have reported a similar ranking for drowning[4-6] where, like Australia, the most common site of childhood drownings is the domestic swimming pool. For each child who drowns, six to nine others are admitted to hospital as a result of a near-drowning incident[3 4 7-9] with 5–20% of these survivors left with permanent brain damage.[4 10]

Numerous studies have indicated that isolating the pool from the house is a successful strategy in reducing the incidence of toddler drowning.[7 11-14] Where immersion incidents do occur in pools with isolation fencing, access was invariably gained through an open or faulty gate or fence, or following parental assistance. Perimeter fencing of a swimming pool addresses less

97

than 3% of child drowning cases, since over 97% of drowned children were already on the property (as residents or invited guests).[7] It has thus been argued that pools should be separated from houses by *isolation* fencing, placing a barrier between the house and the pool. Since the mid-1970s the Child Accident Prevention Foundation of Australia has advocated for legislation for compulsory isolation fencing around all private pools. Sections of the building industry were supportive, perhaps sensing that compulsory fencing would translate into lucrative business, with the average fence costing $4000–5000.[15]

The NSW Swimming Pools Act 1990 was passed, requiring isolation fencing of all new pools. Significantly, it also required that all existing pools be retrospectively isolated by fencing by August 1992. The new law met with considerable opposition from a group of pool owners who formed the PFAG. In the April 1991 State election, the Minister for Local Government who had shepherded the Act through parliament lost his seat amid an unexpected severe general loss of seats by the Liberal/National Government. In September 1991, amid an atmosphere of political scapegoating, it was reported[16] that an internal report to the governing Liberal Party identified the pool fence law as an issue that caused electoral damage to the Government.

The incumbent Minister was adamant from the outset of his Ministry that the pool fencing law would be "reviewed". He established the Pool Fence Review Committee and, in January 1992, the Committee published two reports: a majority report that recommended isolation fencing for all new pools and isolation fencing for existing pools at point of sale or whenever a house was undergoing major renovation; and a minority report that argued for perimeter fencing only. The new Minister supported the minority report.

Framing of debate*

In scientific journals, scholarly policy debates, and the courts, conventions require that issues be expressed in terms of facts and coherent arguments. But as we have argued in previous chapters, in the news media, the demands of brevity and the nature of

* All italicised emphases in press citations are mine.

newsworthiness require that issues be framed through the transformation of facts and arguments into metaphors, labels, and symbols, to allow them to be told as news "stories". In the issue-rich environments of post-industrial societies where many thousands of issues are discussed annually and debated in the mass media by advocates representing different interests, relatively few members of any audience or readership have specialised knowledge of any given issue. Rather, they consume and assess news stories in terms of the values, juxtapositions and framings in which reportage is enmeshed. Public attitudes are shaped by positive and negative symbols that capture and reflect widely shared public values.

In policy disputes requiring public and political support, the media are invariably the battlegrounds on which each side seeks to secure the most powerful positive connotations for its cause, and to attribute to its adversaries the most negative associations. How issues are framed in the media—and how they can be strategically reframed as the prevailing definition of an issue changes—can be highly influential in determining the outcome of an advocacy campaign. This perspective is very relevant to the conduct and interpretation of the pool fencing debate in NSW.

I subjected all Sydney press reports of the pool fencing debate to a discourse analysis. The main themes that emerged from this analysis are discussed here in detail.

Invocation of expertise

It is sometimes naively assumed that political decisions about public health policies result from some objective and meticulous examination of the "facts" surrounding an issue. By this view, those who have the "best" facts will find their arguments treated more sympathetically than those with inferior facts. Plainly, there are many other considerations that often decide the fate of a policy.

Few public debates, however, feature parties who resile completely from attempting to claim possession of the most correct and relevant facts.

In the pool debate, both sides claimed the high ground in expertise. Fence advocates, who were mostly paediatricians, injury prevention epidemiologists and retired judges, had used their data on pool drownings and the common absence of adequate fences as the cornerstone of their advocacy for isolation fencing. Fence opponents thus could hardly avoid engaging with the very basis of the fence policy: that they would supposedly save lives. Here, their strategy was to position the debate as one where experts were in disagreement. For example, a report of a PFAG protest meeting stated: "Pool owners heard *a number of expert speakers* who said [the new regulations] would not make outdoor swimming pools any safer for children" (*North Shore Times*, 30 June 1990). Similarly, a PFAG advertisement summarised an unreferenced "study conducted *by University researchers*" purportedly showing that 20% of three year olds could scale "a 1.2 metre fence in 16 seconds" (*Financial Review*, 25 October 1990) and thus supposedly demonstrating the folly of isolation fencing.

The invocation of expertise by both sides would have promoted a public definition of the facts as having "two sides", thereby allowing politicians to couch the eventual regulation in terms that went beyond an ability to point to any simple right/wrong basis for their judgement.

The populist notions that "there are two sides to every story" and that statistics are inherently suspicious were appropriated candidly by the State Premier when explaining the rejection of the isolation fencing provisions: "You can use facts to support any point of view on this issue, from saying it is entirely a parental responsibility to suggesting that every pool ought to have isolation fencing."[2] The subtext of this statement was: "Don't bother me with factual detail—the facts here are rubbery and cannot be the basis for a policy decision", thus allowing the debate to be resolved through reference to non-factual considerations.

Arguments based on data were also used to try and address the popular support for isolation fencing. The NSW Health Department had conducted a public opinion survey[17] which found that nearly 90% of adults surveyed believed that isolation fencing should be compulsory for all private swimming pools. Most (69%) pool owners who had yet to comply with the legislation also supported it. The report thus was potentially powerful ammunition in showing that isolation fencing had popular support, and that the views of the PFAG were those of an unrepresentative minority.

Accordingly, the PFAG sought to publicly discredit the Report and thereby undermine its relevance to political decision making. Figures in the Report were described as "misleading and inaccurate" and press reports stated somewhat vaguely that it had been "discredited by *at least two senior academics* as being 'methodologically suspect'." A PFAG spokesman said "The fact is that the survey is so flawed as to be useless and indeed a waste of taxpayers' money . . . opinion surveys . . . should be conducted according to the *highest professional criteria*. This survey was not so conducted" (*Sydney Morning Herald*, 12 March 1992).

Although criticisms of the survey had been submitted to the Review Committee, no details of the nature of the Report's alleged problems were reported in the press. The newsworthiness of the criticisms thus lay not in their detail or their veracity, but simply in the fact of their having been made. Fence advocates similarly attacked the factual basis of claims by fence opponents. Arguments about the counterproductivity of fences were said to be a "gross misrepresentation of the facts" (*Sydney Morning Herald* 7 September 1991) and "trumped up to support their own cause" (*Sydney Morning Herald* 31 March 1992). Similarly, the public were not exposed to the nature of the misrepresentations, only to their existence.

Frames used by isolation fence opponents

My home is my castle: the backyard as sanctuary from "Big Brother" government

In Australian urban culture, the backyard is idealised as a distinctly private haven for relaxation and recreation.[18] One's home and backyard are symbolic as a venue for personal freedom and disinhibition. The backyard is a setting for the legitimate expression of an owner's creative impulses promoted and serviced by the gardening, building, and landscaping industries. Here the unruly forces of nature can be tamed and manicured to reflect one's will and good taste. Moreover, the invading forces of the outside world and its laws and preoccupations are held at the arm's length of privacy.

Under the legislation, local government council inspectors would have the right to enter and inspect any premises believed to contain a pool. There are precedents for such entry and inspection that apply to many aspects of domestic conduct (domestic violence, unauthorised building construction, back-yard burning, the unauthorised keeping of poultry or livestock, and cruelty to pet animals). Failure to comply with the legislation would entitle a council to bring in its own contractors to erect a fence at the pool owner's expense. The notion that the Government would be an intrusive, unwelcome presence in this iconic Australian sanctuary was expressed frequently by anti-fence proponents, and was probably the most powerful theme underlying their opposition:

I do object strongly to *Big Brother wanting to come into my backyard and compel me* to do something. (*Sun Herald*, 22 March 1992.)

Isolation fencing is *an invasion* of private residential rights. (*North Shore Times*, 13 July 1990.)

A fascist regime telling people how to look after their children *in their own backyards*. (*Manly Daily*, 26 July 1990.)

Victim blaming

Isolation fencing opponents consistently sought to define pool drownings in terms of parental or supervisory negligence. Put simply, it was said that the parents of drowned children were to blame for their children's deaths.

No-one makes the realistic observation that in nearly every one of these tragic cases *the parent or minder is to blame because of careless and inadequate supervision*. (*Sydney Morning Herald*, 18 November 1989.)

These are obviously *people who don't know how to look after their children*. (*Weekend Australian*, 1–2 September 1990.)

A fence should not be made the guardian of our children . . . It's *only responsible supervision that saves children's lives*. (*Manly Daily*, 26 July 1990.)

Eternal vigilance with little ones is the only way we can minimise child accidents. (*Sydney Morning Herald*, 27 March 1992.)

Significantly, the Premier, in explaining his Government's decision to accept the minority (anti-isolation fencing) report of the Review Committee, invoked this frame and embellished it with the language of corporate managerialism that had characterised his Government's overall philosophy: "You can't legislate against irresponsible human behaviour . . . more than half of all toddler deaths occur because *human beings haven't managed to manage their back yards properly*" (*Sydney Morning Herald*, 7 April 1992).

Drowning as punishment for trespass

The frame of blaming the victim was extended by one writer to become a definition of victim punishment. Following the suggestion by a rebel Government supporter of isolation fences that small children who wandered into neighbours' gardens and drowned in their pools were having "the death penalty imposed for trespassing" ("More than 30% of children who drown in pools are uninvited. Why should we impose the death penalty on young children for trespassing?" (*North Shore Times*, 30 June 1990)), a citizen replied: "Whatever happened to 'enter at own risk'? Or are we too concerned with *protecting the criminal element* of our society. Then again, why not make it compulsory to have big foam cushions mounted on the front of all buses and cars as a safety precaution [against knocking down children]" (*North Shore Times*, 13 July 1990).

Fences as counterproductive

Fence opponents argued that, rather than preventing drownings, isolation fences would actually cause more drownings by replacing parental vigilance with indifference. The subtext of this argument was thus: "You want us to sleep with the enemy. The very thing you say we should trust will kill our children." "By bringing in this new fencing law, parents are going to be *lulled into a false sense of security*." (*Manly Daily*, 26 July 1990).

One letter writer perhaps unwittingly acknowledged that unfenced pools would result in immersion "emergencies", but chose to interpret this as an argument against fences, reasoning that a successful rescue was preferable to preventing the need for a rescue in the first place: "We believe it is safer to have instant access to pools *for emergencies*" (*North Shore Times*, 13 July 1990).

Arbitrary fencing of (pool) water as capricious folly

The PFAG adapted a common argument frequently resorted to by interest groups seeking to avoid their activities being controlled: if you can't eliminate all problems, don't try to eliminate any of them. The PFAG pointed out that there are many water sources where children drown which are neither fenced, nor planned to be. Hence, fencing only swimming pools was argued to be capricious, arbitrary, and thus supposedly revealing of the Government's lack of real resolve to reduce drowning. It was rather some ill conceived knee-jerk reaction.

Are there fences around ponds in parks, dams on farms etc? (*Sydney Morning Herald*, 18 November 1989.)

Children are drowning in buckets, dams, stormwater drains, rivers and creeks . . . yet *the Government has chosen to ignore these deaths* even though they exceed drownings in private pools. (*Financial Review*, 25 October 1990.)

Hysteria and emotional claptrap

Isolation fence advocates were depicted as hysterical, illogical, and proponents of "emotional claptrap", with the obvious subtext that rational, cool-headed, Government decision making should not be influenced by the ravings of such people.

Every unfortunate time a small child drowns in a pool there is *hysteria* by the Minister for Local Government. (*Sydney Morning Herald*, 18 November 1989.)

These are *people who have lost all logic*. (*Weekend Australian*, 1–2 September 1990.)

The Government was led up the garden path by *emotional claptrap*. (*Glebe and Western Weekly*, 12 September 1990.)

When the Government overturned the isolation fencing requirement, the PFAG declared, "We are happy that there has been *some genuine commonsense* brought into this debate" (*Sydney Morning Herald*, 2 April 1992).

Overkill

The 1990 law required that all pools would need isolation fencing. The PFAG sought to highlight examples of people who never had children in their pools as exemplifying why this blanket provision in the law was draconian overkill: like the Government using a sledgehammer to crack a walnut. Citing distressed pensioners who would allegedly be severely financially hurt by having to erect a fence seemed an attempt to evoke a view of the Government as both irrationally stubborn and heartless: "We've had calls from pensioners . . . who don't even have children in their pools" (*Manly Daily*, 26 July 1990). "I've had [pensioners] *crying on the phone to me*" (*Weekend Australian*, 1–2 September 1990).

Authentic, committed citizens versus paid civil servants

Throughout the debate, fence advocates sought to portray fence opponents as affluent, selfish, and lacking compassion for drowning victims and their parents (see below). Advocates for isolation fences were almost exclusively medical practitioners and researchers (and sometimes parents of drowned children). Despite swimming pools costing many thousands of dollars to build and maintain and the PFAG being concentrated in Sydney's affluent North Shore region, the PFAG sought to reframe themselves as ordinary, often impoverished, citizens and their foes as people unwilling to finance their convictions through their own pockets. The subtext of these frames was that fence opponents were authentic, personally committed, and genuine, while fence advocates were by comparison inauthentic and so not as credible. "[Our] funds came from ordinary pool owners, many of whom were pensioners or unemployed . . . Unlike the pro-fencing lobby, we have had no-one paid an income from the public purse to run our campaign" (*Sydney Morning Herald*, 2 July 1992).

Fence opponents were undoubtedly partly motivated by concern about the costs of erecting fences, but equally concerned to emphasise that their opposition had nothing to do with their being parsimonious: "It's a lot of money to fork out and nobody would mind if this was a sure way of stopping drownings" (*Manly Daily*, 26 July 1990).

Frames used by isolation fence advocates

Personalising: the human face of infant drowning

Fence opponents generally avoided discussing particular drowning incidents, preferring to refer to deaths in the abstract, perfectly illustrated by a letter writer who wrote of the argument for fences: "In order to stop *someone's hypothetical child*" from drowning (*Sydney Morning Herald*, 27 March 1992). Fence advocates countered by seeking to put a human face on such abstractions, with one advocate's press letter describing a public meeting he had attended:

Whenever toddler deaths were talked about *in real human terms rather than just numbers,* the *speakers were met with snickering, jeers* and calls of "that's an emotional argument". Well, this is an emotional issue. Trying to resuscitate a drowning child, or telling the parents that their child has died is *a sad, tragic, emotional experience.* (*Sydney Morning Herald*, 7 September 1991.)

Feature articles on victim profiles were also published which detailed the consequences of immersion and families' anguish: "Thomas Rennick lived for 15 months, unable to see, hear, speak, feel or move. For months, he was fed with a nasal-gastric tube until he recovered his swallowing reflex, and he finally died in his sleep" (*Weekend Australian*, 1–2 September 1990).

Parents as fallible, human

Attempts were made to reframe the parental responsibility, victim-blaming definition of infant drowning in terms of the sheer unreasonableness of the view that parents could ever be constantly vigilant: "You can't look after your child *every hour, every minute of every day*" (*Sydney Morning Herald*, 31 March 1992) and "This is why we need to employ safety measures that cannot be distracted, such as isolation fences" (*Sydney Morning Herald*, 7 September 1991).

Aesthetics versus saving a child's life

Pro-fence advocates sought to depict their opponents' objections as founded on a "smokescreen of rights and aesthetics"

(*Sydney Morning Herald*, 27 March 1993) and the Government's 1992 capitulation as "appeas[ing] a *selfish minority* group who were *more concerned with their backyard aesthetics and their civil rights than child safety*" (*Sydney Morning Herald*, 31 March 1992). "Some people see a fence as an affront and an architectural blunder that they don't need" (*Manly Daily*, 25 October 1989).

In an editorial, the view that a child's life was priceless was invoked in apposition to the ephemeral values of convenience and glamour. "People who want the convenience and glamour of a swimming pool must also be prepared to accept the responsibility and costs associated with reducing the danger of drownings in that pool. It may cost around $4,000 to install an isolation fence, but a child's life is priceless" (*Newcastle Herald*, 7 April 1992).

Inconsistency with existing safety standards

The fence opponents' frame of "Big Brother" government intruding into homes with expensive, outrageous demands was countered by advocates listing precedents for mandatory safety measures in homes: "Electrical safety, stairs, fire escapes, balustrade construction" (*Sydney Morning Herald*, 7 September 1991). Here were examples of imposed, mandatory and sometimes expensive requirements that the state required of private home owners for reasons that were seldom, if ever, challenged as being draconian imposts on individual freedom. Ought not pool fences be seen in the same light, the analogy begged? A different inflexion of this theme was expressed by a letter writer who argued, "A pool fence is like compulsory third party insurance. If you can't afford the insurance you can't afford the car" (*Sydney Morning Herald*, 27 March 1992). A parent, being interviewed on a television programme, argued alliteratively: "If you can't afford the fence, you can't afford the funeral."

One fence advocate stated, "If a bus crashed and that many kids were killed, we would have instant action" (*Sydney Morning Herald*, 15 November 1989). This undoubtedly correct assessment, however, obviated one of the essential problems that the fence advocates faced: the 10 children who on average drowned in NSW pools each year would never all die in a mass drowning in the one pool; they died alone, scattered throughout the state, thereby allowing a dissipation of the community outrage that would have surely followed a mass drowning.

A vocal, selfish minority

Fence opponents were continually described as small in number (*Sydney Morning Herald*, 5 April 1991), a "vocal minority" (*Sydney Morning Herald*, 7 September 1991) and a group who were affluent and had access to the Government: "This is a victory for a *very small, very vocal* and obviously very influential group of pool owners with *plenty of funds* to wage their campaign and with *very good access to senior ministers*" (*Sydney Morning Herald*, 2 July 1992). The Government was accused of "outrageous kowtowing" to this group (*Sydney Morning Herald*, 25 March 1992). It was reported that a key member of the PFAG was a former President of the NSW Liberal Party.

Votes versus children's lives

When the Government sought to explain their decision to rescind isolation fencing requirements in terms of a combination of promoting parental responsibility and being unconvinced by the evidence on fence protectiveness, fence advocates attempted to reframe their motivation in terms of "The Government has obviously made a political decision. They have listened to a small but vocal minority, most of whom . . . live in Liberal seats" (*Sydney Morning Herald*, 2 April 1992). When the Opposition Labor Party dropped its support of fences, the advocates' response was similar: "If politicians want to seek votes at the expense of children's lives, then I think that is deplorable" (*Sydney Morning Herald*, 5 April 1991).

Defenders of the innocent and helpless

Attempts were made to position pool advocacy arguments as giving a voice to children too young and powerless to have a say in a matter that would affect their lives. The civil liberties' argument of fence opponents was appropriated in service of this new definition, "any measure that will reduce the tragic deaths of toddlers is in fact upholding the civil liberties of *those too young to demand them for themselves"* (*Sydney Morning Herald*, 7 September 1991).

Discussion

Our analysis shows that public debate centred around struggles for dominance in five main areas of argument, summarised in Table VI. We believe the following "deep structural" oppositions finally characterised the two groups' positions.

Fence proponents

The pro-fence group positioned themselves as advocates for the protection of the lives of small children, an almost inviolate moral high ground in virtually every society, and therefore an enormously powerful starting point. They consistently implied that to value any other consideration such as votes, garden aesthetics, and the avoidance of a financial outlay (especially by those affluent enough to have a private pool), above a commitment to saving children's lives, was the moral equivalent of infanticide. Having commenced the debate, the pro-fence advocates were on the offensive from the beginning, although soon found themselves on the defensive in the face of their opponent's frames.

Fence opponents

For fence opponents, this was a formidable definition of the issue and one that required a distracting, powerful reframing. They astutely elected also to inhabit the pro-fence frame ("We also want to save children's lives") but to argue that the fence advocates were dangerously misguided: their emotionalism had blinded them to the real cause of drowning (negligent, "bad" parenting) and the counterproductivity of their isolation fence solution. In these emphases, fencing opponents displayed an identical range of ideological and rhetorical arguments to those used by opponents of fences in Queensland between 1976 and 1978, as reported in a study of letters to the Editors of various Queensland newspapers.[19]

Most significantly, they were also able to embed their oppo-

Table VI: Arguments of pool fencing advocates and opponents

Area of argument	Fencing advocates' framings	Fencing opponents' framings
Why pool drownings occur	Children are naturally inquisitive, exploratory It is human for parental vigilance to be fallible Some drownings are unsighted "trespassing" children	Parental negligence; bad parenting Trespassers should be given little sympathy; blame the victim
The effects of fencing and non-fencing	Will prevent unsupervised access, reduce immersion and drownings—the evidence shows it Child drownings as tragic, justifiably "emotional" Personalisation: here are the real victims of drownings behind the statistics	Fences will increase parental complacency and drownings Statistical improbability of a drowning in any one pool ("some hypothetical child") They are using a sledgehammer to crack a walnut
Expert views, community support	Experts are united in support of fences Survey shows community strongly supportive	Our experts say your conclusions are unjustified Your community opinion survey flawed, worthless
The role of the state in prevention	There are many imposed, often costly, safety precedents A child's life is priceless Children's lives are more important than winning votes Protecting its citizens (especially those who can't protect themselves) *is* an important role for the state	Our homes are our castles; sanctuary from "Big Brother" government A universal fencing requirement will needlessly hurt those with no children, especially pensioners Fencing only pools is capricious folly when other waterways remain accessible
Who are we/they?	We are defenders of the innocent and voiceless Our only concern is with child safety—we have no other vested interests We are unashamedly emotional about the preventable tragedy of child drownings They value garden aesthetics more than a child's life They are a vocal, selfish, rich, influential minority They are parsimonious; want the pleasure of a pool without the responsibility of fencing it	We are anti-"Big Brother" government We are primarily concerned with child safety—but they have the wrong solution They are emotional, illogical, hysterical We fund our own opposition to the policy/they don't have the financial courage of their convictions

sition to fences in an ideological reference system that placed them as natural allies with the conservative Government. In its shared espousal of a non-interventionist political philosophy and a preoccupation about individual responsibility (drownings result from negligent parenting), the PFAG's arguments would have been more consonant with the values of the Government than the essentially state-interventionist, regulatory position central to the pro-fence policy. The polarisation of the two lobbies reflected a critical ideological difference between those who support interventionist policies, which sometimes regulate the freedoms of individuals to protect or enhance the public benefit, and those who believe that individuals should fend for themselves.

The passage of the 1990 Act was almost certainly a function of an organised isolation fence advocacy campaign conducted under the support of a Government Minister who was personally dedicated to the cause, in the face of protests by a (then) unorganised opposition. The intervening period (1990–2) was notably different. While fence advocates inflexibly maintained their demands, the other two factors changed considerably.

What lessons are there for advocates of isolation fencing in this case study? In hindsight, they may well have seriously misread how onerous the costs of fencing appeared to pool owners. In the 1990 Act, isolation fence advocates had succeeded in having an extremely radical piece of legislation passed. Although there had been precedents of retrospective safety legislation in recent Australian social life—for example, front and, later, rear seat car belts; motorcycle and bicycle helmets), each of these examples had required consumers to outlay relatively small amounts of money compared with the costs of erecting isolation fencing. There was simply no precedent for safety legislation that required an across the board retrospective and prospective financial outlay of such proportions. This core aspect of the isolation fencing proposal clearly galvanised a degree of opposition that might otherwise have been much less.

The retrospective fencing demand seems likely to have been the principal feature of the legislation that would have motivated considerable animosity among pool owners. Had the original 1990 Act required only prospective isolation fencing (at times of house sale or pool installation), it is probable that much of the vehemence in the opposition to fences would have been neutralised. Prospective fencing would have passed on both the cost and aesthetic disadvantages, and the very consideration of the issue, to future pool owners. It seems highly unlikely that many people merely either imminently or distantly *considering* buying a house with a pool or building a pool would have anything remotely like the same emotional investment in the fencing debate.

Prospective fencing would have almost certainly met with feeble opposition, but would have represented a compromise on the objective of having all pools fenced as quickly as possible. The Majority Report of the Government's Pool Fence Review Committee recommended that pools be fenced prospectively (either at pool installation or at point of sale of the house). The failure of the pro-fence lobby to have advocated this approach in the initial legislation of 1990 resulted in the rise of a vociferous opposition and the eventual acceptance by the Government of the minority report, the recommendations of which were less acceptable to the fence advocates than those (prospective) compromises recommended by the majority report.

The refusal to compromise on the issue of retrospective fencing reflected their assumption that the only acceptable number of infant drownings was zero: it was as if while there were *any* drownings, there could never be any question of compromising on fences. In recent years, the average annual number of infant pool drownings in NSW has been about 10. Fence advocates clearly regarded this number as wholly unacceptable, while fence opponents appeared to be complacent about such a figure. They argued that the 10 annual drownings meant a 1 in 20 000 chance of a drowning occurring in any one of the state's 200 000 pools, or more dramatically that "a child would drown in any particular pool once every 21 000 years"[20] was an acceptable price to pay for the freedom not to fence all pools. While the probability of a drowning occurring in any one pool in a given year is remote, the probability dramatically increases over the lifetime of a pool, particularly if fenced pools were removed from the calculation. Far more dramatic purpose could have been made of such a calculation.

Finally, the resistance to the fence opponents' criticisms of the community opinion survey (which overwhelmingly showed public support for mandatory fencing) was weak. In large part this was because the survey was commissioned by Government employees in the Health Department. These people were placed in an awkward position of being unable to defend their survey vigorously because of their (the Government) employer's own agenda which seemed intent on diluting the 1990 Act. The lesson here is that, in such circumstances, such research needs to be conducted by independent community or academic groups who are uncompromised in their ability to defend their work.

Case study 2: anatomy of a campaign—the attempt to defeat the NSW Tobacco Advertising Prohibition Bill, 1991

Background

As a result of national government legislation, direct advertising of cigarettes has been prohibited on Australian radio and television since 1976 and in locally published print media since December 1990. The remaining forms of advertising (cinema, outdoor, sampling, shopfront, and point of sale) are under the control of each of the six State and two Territory Governments. In the past five years, four of these have legislated to prohibit these remaining forms that fell under their jurisdiction. New South Wales (NSW) is the most populous state and has a conservative (Liberal/National coalition) government in power. Until passage of the NSW Tobacco Advertising Prohibition Bill (1991), outdoor, taxiback, shopfront and point of sale cigarette advertising remained in NSW. These forms will all be phased out by the end of 1995. Massive media coverage also continues to be given to tobacco sponsored events such as the Winfield Rugby League Cup and the international Benson and Hedges cricket series. These two sports dominate (respectively) winter and summer broadcast media sports coverage, regularly heading all other programmes in television audience share ratings. NSW has been widely regarded as symbolic of the industry's last stand in Australia and has enjoyed the overt support of the State Premier who has often publicly trivialised the tobacco control issue, for example, saying recently, that it was "really very marginal to the well-being of mankind."[21]

In 1991, minor political parties and independent politicians held the balance of power in both the Upper and Lower Houses of Parliament in NSW. One such member, Christian fundamentalist, the Reverend Fred Nile, introduced the Tobacco Advertising Prohibition Bill, 1991 which sought to end all remaining forms of tobacco advertising in NSW, including publicity given to sporting sponsorships. Nile had the support of the Opposition (Labor) and Democrat Parties. Together, these groups had the numbers to defeat the Government, which initially indicated that it was vehemently opposed to the Bill. As the date approached for the parliamentary debate, the Government, realising the inevitability of defeat, changed its position and introduced exemption amendments (see below) while executing a *volte face* and declaring that it now supported the overall thrust of the Bill to ban all remaining forms of advertising.[22]

When Nile's intentions became public, the tobacco industry, through its lobby office, the Tobacco Institute, launched a huge press advertising campaign in an attempt to scare away political support in all parties from the Bill. Sporting groups receiving tobacco sponsorship also supported the industry campaign through lobbying, advertising, and media announcements. The size and ferocity of the campaign were testimony to the degree of concern the industry felt at the prospects of losing the remainder of its advertising outlets and of a possible boost to an international domino effect. Grand hyperbole frequently ran riot in the advertising with claims such as: the politicians behind the ban were "effectively running our state and our lives. This is only the start of what he has in mind for us. Books and alcohol are firm favourites!"

The principal themes and rhetorical devices used in the industry campaign are described below. These exhibit several approaches long favoured by the industry in its international lobbying. Several significant emphases and admissions emerged, however, which will interest all who are concerned to keep abreast of the industry's tactics in this field. Given the sheer volume of advertising published, examples have been extracted of the themes under various headings, rather than attempting any exhaustive catalogue of all that was run by the industry and its supporters. My emphases are italicised throughout.

Enough is enough

One theme, encapsulated in the repeated headline: "Enough is enough!" dominated the campaign. This was shorthand for a complex connotative chain evoking notions of unfairness, bullying, lack of compassion, and of Orwellian government lawmakers running out of control ("Any politicians who support the Bill are displaying *a callous disregard for the welfare of the ordinary people* of NSW", argued one ad.). Akin to the proverbial "slippery slope", "thin end of the wedge", or "where will it all end?" rhetoric long favoured by the industry, the slogan sat astride advertisements ranging from cartoons mocking the politicians who supported the Bill, to testimonial advertising from sponsored sporting groups, allied industries (for example, printing) and "little people" said to be about to suffer at the hand of the Bill's provisions. Subthemes under the "Enough is Enough" banner included the following.

Jobs will be lost

The proposed ban may well have caused some job losses in, for example, advertising agencies which would have lost tobacco accounts, and in poster hanging companies which have in recent years benefited greatly from restrictions in other tobacco advertising outlets. It would have been difficult, however, for the industry to argue that these losses would number scarcely more than 100 in NSW. As such, there was about as much capital in arguing for the retention of these jobs as the motor vehicle repair industry complaining about lost jobs due to the downturn in road crashes caused by the introduction of random alcohol breath testing (as indeed some newspaper letter writers did, tongue in cheek, during the campaign).

Faced with this situation, the industry threw all caution to the wind with claims of job losses right across the tobacco spectrum. Despite its usual meticulous insistence that advertising does not influence aggregate demand for cigarettes, any pretence that the proposed ban would *not* cause a downturn in sales was utterly abandoned in this campaign. The Tobacco Institute claimed that the Bill "puts at risk the livelihoods of 25 344 other decent Australians who make their living from the tobacco industry in NSW. There are growers, manufacturers, shop floor, wholesalers, retailers, drivers, packers, not to mention the printers, shop fitters, painters, outdoor advertising companies and their sales staff." Similar claims were made by the tobacco retailers' trade association, which argued that restrictions on even point of sale advertising threatened to "ultimately result in . . . the loss of another 25 000 jobs in the long term . . . hundreds of resellers [retailers] will eventually go out of business." The printing industry, which prints advertising signs and cigarette packs, claimed, "If this is done in NSW, jobs will be lost—and some printing companies will be forced to close their doors because of the millions of dollars of revenue that is at risk in our industry alone."

The logic of these claims bordered on the asinine with internally contradictory claims such as the Bill would "reduce the number of jobs in this State rather than the incidence of smoking" and *"Banning advertising won't stop people smoking.* But the minority think differently. *They want us to sacrifice jobs,* funds for sport, and the arts, *for an idea which doesn't work.* Don't let their minority opinions overthrow plain common sense." Here it can be seen that "common sense" to the industry means the ability to contradict oneself totally within one sentence: if advertising bans won't reduce smoking, how is it that jobs could be lost?

Hardship for the "little" person during the recession

Several advertisements featured owners of small businesses who would allegedly suffer financial hardship if the advertising ban was enacted. Advertisements entitled: "Don't kick us while we're down" featured testimonials from an outdoor poster hanger:

"I wish the politicians would listen to *the little people* before they start bringing in new Bills! I reckon contractors stand to lose roughly $500 a week if the Anti-Tobacco Bill goes through . . . The tobacco companies spend millions on outdoor advertising. You simply can't take that much out of an industry and not lose jobs! It's no use saying other people will take the space . . . So here we go again. The little guys cop it in the neck and politicians wonder why voters are looking for alternatives."

Despite this poster hanger claiming that alternative poster

advertisers would not be available to replace the lost tobacco advertising, in the very same advertisement, in the very next testimonial, a taxi fleet manager seemed to know differently. Speaking of the revenue he got from taxiback tobacco advertising ("It's used to pay my mortgage and general bills"), he said "Believe me in this recession it's not easy to get advertisers . . . The big advertisers will be *busy taking over the big outdoor contracts currently held by tobacco companies*. They won't be interested in taxis. It's the little people who will get hurt, again!"

A country town tobacconist claimed the Bill "means I'll have to refit my shop inside and out so people can't see any tobacco advertising." In fact all the typical tobacconist would have to do would be to peel off stick-on advertising from windows, remove cardboard advertisements from display areas and perhaps paint over signage. Given that there was a phase out period of four years for this provision of the Bill, the tobacconist's complaint suggested a level of interior decorating indolence bordering on the comatose.

Turning decent citizens into "common criminals"

One day before the Bill was due to be debated finally in the Lower House of the Parliament, an advertisement was published headlined:

"Your local newsagent doesn't want to be *made a common criminal* by your local member." Pictured behind superimposed bars were a smiling, middle-aged couple behind the counter of their (named) suburban newsagency. In quotation marks beneath the photo, the couple told readers: "Newsagents are *honest, hardworking small business people*. The new Anti-Tobacco Bill will make it illegal to advertise, on the outside of our shop, which cigarette brands we sell. If there is *even* one cigarette sign outside we could be fined up to $5,000 for the first offence, and then up to $10,000 for a second offence. If we cannot pay we might face jail. Surely the Government and the Opposition have *more important things to do than threaten our livelihoods* with *crippling* penalties. They *should spend more time in the real world* where *making a dollar* is harder than ever before. Now they want to make it even harder. It's OK for them to make 100s of millions in taxes from smokers in NSW—how come it is going to be illegal for us to have cigarette signs

117

on our own shop? It's a *double standard*. We don't want to be *common criminals*. Please let your local member of Parliament know what you think of our *freedom being eroded.*"

Like the earlier "Don't Kick Us While We're Down" advertisement, here was an attempt to show the face of ordinary Australians said to be affected by the Bill. These were "your local newsagents", not anonymous workers in some obscure, dubious section of the tobacco industry. These people looked and sounded uncomplicated, decent, and law abiding. Here were archetypes of the very ordinariness and, above all, reasonableness that the industry wanted to portray as being behind those who wanted to retain tobacco advertising. As owners of small businesses, as distinct from giant corporations, they sought to represent the human face of the consequences of an allegedly ridiculous law. As they say, they are in the *real world*, the corollary of which is that anyone taking a different view is out of touch, a zealot, or a fanatic. Those supporting the Bill were thus marginalised as a discrete "movement". "Consider the views of those outside the anti tobacco movement", urged one advertisement.

The central proposition of this advertisement—that decent, ordinary shopkeepers would be turned into criminals by the passage of the Bill—implied that such shopkeepers would defy the law by continuing to display cigarette advertising. The sheer unlikelihood of this was of course not countenanced by the advertisement. There have been no overt instances of radio, television, or print media defiance of their respective advertising bans.

Hypocrisy

The accusation that there was rank hypocrisy involved in Government collecting tobacco excise taxes while denying the right of sporting groups to accept sponsorship was another common theme. The country tobacconist who complained about his spurious shop refit argued: "Yet the Government will still collect the revenue on the cigarettes I sell. They don't seem to care if I can't find the money for the refit. So as the business dies, after years of building it up, I'll have to start putting off temporary staff and eventually loyal permanent staff. Our politicians should explain the true repercussions of this bill to these people."

The accusation of "hypocrisy" was countered in responses from the Bill's protagonists by reference to tobacco use contributing to the costs of public health care for diseases caused by smoking, and thereby seeking to deny that there was any moral equivalence between Government being allowed to take tobacco money, but sport being forbidden. But while the industry could lead with its accusations of hypocrisy in full page advertisements and through sympathetic media sports commentators, the counterview could only be put out by politicians and health authorities in news releases and opportunist media interviews.

Neo-puritanism or "wowserism"

The Reverend Fred Nile who introduced the Bill represents the Call to Australia Party, a small party representing "family" values. Nile's main profile before his tobacco Bill had been on anti-abortion and anti-homosexual law reform issues, and in his attempts to remove books with sexual scenes and "bad language" from school libraries. In each of these areas he had been spectacularly unsuccessful and had been pilloried and openly mocked throughout the liberal media. On his announcement of the Bill, however, the gay lobby announced that the Bill was "the only anti-fag legislation it would ever support."[23]

Nile's carriage of the Bill into Parliament was like oxygen to the flame of puritanism, a theme that the tobacco industry has often sought to nurture in its characterisation of those seeking to restrict its activities. Nile provided his opponents with a set of gift wrapped, negative appositions they sought to exploit in several advertisements, including a cartoon clearly designed to offend Nile, which showed him naked in bed with a disconcerted Leader of the Opposition, suggesting that their political collusion on this issue had wider implications.

"Wowser" is a colloquial Australian term meaning "a censorious person, a killjoy"[24] and is commonly applied to anyone who seeks to suppress pleasure or fun. Historically, the term has been applied to the alcohol temperance movement, to those offended by public nudity or brief swimwear, and, lately, to people concerned about smoking. A cartoon advertisement headed

NSWowser showed Nile addressing a crowd with the words: "No smoking, drinking, swearing, no adult books or videos . . . no topless bathing . . . no horses, trots or greyhounds . . . no casinos, TAB [licensed betting], lotteries or scratch-cards . . . But I have arranged for cucumber sandwiches and tea and lamingtons [an Australian cake popular with older people] prior to 6 o'clock [bar] closing." The advertisement concluded: "Is this the sort of NSW we want to live in?"

Freedom to choose

The NSW Rugby League, whose game is sponsored by the Winfield brand, ran an advertisement focusing on their right to choose any sponsor and describing this as almost a nationalist duty: "As Australians we have a history of standing up for our rights. It's one of the great things that makes us Australian." Another continued in the same vein: "Is this the freedom our parents and grandparents fought for?"

An advertisement titled "The world according to Fred Nile (and all the other wowsers in the NSW parliament)" sought to obfuscate the objectives of the Bill, suggesting that Nile was attempting to ban smoking. Captioned against a series of cartoon characters it read: "I like to drive a car, I take the gamble, I like to over-eat, I take the gamble. I like to mountain-climb, I take the gamble. I like to race motor bikes, I take the gamble. I like to chase cars, I take the gamble [a talking dog]." The cartoon ended with Nile saying, "I like to make choices for everyone else, and I don't agree with gambling!" It concluded, "We want the right to choose our own adult recreations"—as if sport or smoking itself were to be banned under the legislation.

Another stated, "If the Bill is passed, it will make it illegal for sporting groups to freely choose their own sponsors." Again, this was gross obfuscation: sporting groups would remain free to choose any sponsor, including a tobacco company, providing the tobacco company was prepared to forgo the publicity that sponsorships traditionally entail. A host of large corporations were described in the press as likely to be interested in sponsoring the main tobacco sponsored sports such as cricket and rugby.

One advertisement ambiguously suggested that the Bill would ban sponsorship *per se*, rather than tobacco sponsorship. Its headline read that the Bill "will ban the sponsorship of the Winfield Cup [rugby league] and horse races, B&H World Series Cricket and Skiing, Peter Jackson motor racing, Rothmans bike racing and rugby union and the Philip Morris Arts Grant and Superband."

Paternalism

Related to the freedom issue was the theme of the proposed law and the political climate which spawned it as being paternalistic. "Australian adults are NOT children", argued one. "We must let all politicians know we are adults and we want to do what we like when we like—within the law" said another. While politicians are elected to represent the people and to enact legislative reform, this point seemed lost on the industry: "Fred Nile thinks he knows what is best for all of us", it argued, as if Nile had no business attempting to pursue his mandate.

Surveys of public opinion

The industry commissioned several "surveys" and published the results in advertisements with titles such as "Listen to the people". The surveys were somewhat biased, one starting with the question: "As a non smoker do you think tobacco companies sponsoring sporting events, the arts and concerts is likely or unlikely to make you take up smoking?" With the predictability of day following night, 98% of respondents answered "unlikely". By asking this question first, a response bias was introduced that influenced subsequent, less loaded questions, all of which predictably went the industry's way.

Easily the most controversial "poll" result followed an advertisement placed by the NSW Cricket Association titled "Don't let the lights go out on cricket." This invited readers to call a toll-free phone number and register their opposition to the Bill. Callers supporting the Bill would not have their votes registered by this process. Yet, despite this, an advertisement published three days later and authorised by the Tobacco Institute, reported 90% of callers to be in favour and 10% to be against. When confronted with this apparent discrepancy by a television reporter the ensuing dialogue took place on ABC's 7.30 Report:

121

John Welch (Tobacco Institute): That was the result.

Interviewer: But they were only taking the "no" votes, you must have known that?

Welch: I did not have anything to do with that survey . . . other than advised of the result.

Interviewer: But by running that statistic, you're misinforming the public. Would you concede that it might have been ill advised for you to run that figure?

Welch: I've told you, I don't concede anything. This is a battle and you never take a backward step.

No advertising in Russia

An advertisement titled "Most Russians have never seen a cigarette ad, so how come they smoke more than us?" explained to readers:

In Russia, where cigarette advertising hasn't been allowed for over sixty years, more than double the percentage of the population smoke compared to Australians. What makes them start? Quite obviously it isn't advertising or sponsorship. A State run tobacco monopoly doesn't need it. In Australia a vocal minority keep arguing that cigarette advertising makes non-smokers start smoking. Clearly, countries like Russia and many others show this theory is rubbish.

Correspondents to newspapers replied that cigarettes were one of the few consumer goods readily available in the USSR; that they were extremely cheap; and that widespread health promotion campaigns did not exist. Still, the complexities of the arguments about the causal relationship between advertising and consumption[25] are almost certainly less resonant and persuasive to many people than the simplistic appeal of the argument put out by the industry.

Discussion

The industry's campaign failed to deter politicians from passing the Bill, although a major amendment which was accepted (allowing sports with "national or international significance" to seek exemption from the phased out sponsorship ban from the

Government) means that this issue remains far from resolved in Australia. This exemption means that any NSW government sympathetic to the industry has the discretion to allow a high profile sport to continue its very public association with the industry. Federal (Labor) Ministers for Health and Sport have already announced their intention to close this loophole through amendments to national broadcast legislation which would override any State's actions in this area. The political configuration—the hung Parliament with a majority supporting the Bill—that existed in NSW meant that the Bill would inevitably pass, even without the support of the Government, so it is interesting to speculate on why the industry spent the millions of dollars it did on the campaign.

The power of its starting arsenal was obvious: money and many grateful beneficiaries willing to do the industry's bidding. As it is not permitted to advertise in the most expensive media (broadcast and print), the industry has by default become a gargantuan advertiser in the outdoor and shopfront media, providing expensive shop awnings, table umbrellas and lucrative display incentives to owners of small shops. Similarly in sport, its advertising reserves are such that it has been able to offer sponsorships at premium levels way above the market rates negotiated by other commercial sponsors. If an oil company and a car company (which have other direct advertising options) were competitively negotiating sponsorship with a sport around a figure of, say, $2 million, tobacco companies in Australia could offer unparalleled higher sums. For example, in 1988, the Winfield Rugby League sponsorship in NSW was worth only $1.1 million. By 1990 and despite a recessionary environment, this had risen to $8 million,[26] far ahead of estimates for other sponsored sports. Anticipating the advance of further advertising restrictions, the industry has poured rivers of money into sporting sponsorship to a point where most sporting administrators see the prospect of alternative lesser sponsorships as comparative penury.

Thus, beyond its traditional support base of direct beneficiaries (tobacco growers, tobacco workers, and some advertising agencies) the industry has been able to mesmerise some other important constituencies with its artificially high funds. Partial advertising bans in Australia have in this way had the untoward effect of artificially strengthening the bond between the industry and those who are legally still able to promote cigarettes. The emoluments and fringe benefits of sponsorship so vividly documented by Peter Taylor[27] create a dependency among beneficiaries who understandably don't want to kill the goose that lays the golden eggs for the sake of what they hope they can portray as a muddle headed and dubious appeal to public health.

Presumably, the industry had great confidence in the power of its sheer financial clout and in the weight of numbers among its grateful new constituents in small business and sport. The Rugby League, for example, threatened to campaign among its hundreds of thousands of working class, traditionally Labor voting club members, for a political vote against the Opposition Labor party at the next elections.[28] When the Government supported the Bill, this threat became even more lame, with voters having no one now to offer their vote. The themes I have described above were nearly all linked to the consequences that would befall such ordinary Australians going about the pursuit of their incomes and sports. While the proponents of the Bill attempted to frame the meaning of the Bill in terms of public health and the protection of children, the industry sought all but completely to avoid these issues and instead to reframe the issues it judged as serving its interests in the ways we have described.

The most important question that remains is whether, had political support for the Bill been more tenuous, the industry's efforts would have won out. Attempts to answer this question in this instance must remain speculative, but the subject area represents a very neglected field of research in tobacco control. Massive propaganda offensives by the tobacco industry have the potential to undermine both efforts to achieve important legislative reforms in tobacco control and advances in public opinion conducive to reduced smoking. Yet, as an area for serious research, analysis, and strategic development, it remains mysteriously marginalised in the professional literature on tobacco control.

In the opinion of my colleagues in Australia, the most animated discussions appeared to be dominated by the illogical and inept arguments put forward by the industry. Many letters scoring points were written to the press by such people, demonstrating the folly involved and attempting ridicule. Such preoccupations, however, may well be beside the point. Political battles are seldom won only on the elegance of logic or by those who can best assemble rational arguments. These are mere strategies within a wider battle front. The real issue is which are the overall framings of debates that best succeed in capturing public opinion and political will.

References

1 Greiner N. Pool fencing laws protect kids. *North Shore Times* 1990 Jun 30.
2 Garcia LM. Pool fence compromise approved by Cabinet. *Sydney Morning Herald* 1992 May 1.
3 Carey V. Preventing drowning in toddlers. *Injury Issues* (NSW Department of Health) 1991; July 2.
4 Wintemute GJ, Drake C. Immersion events in residential swimming pools. *Am J Dis Child* 1991; **145**: 1200–3.
5 Rowe MI, Arango A, Allington G. Profile of pediatric drowning victims in a water-oriented society. *J Trauma* 1977; **17**: 587–91.
6 Gardiner SD, Smeeton WM, Koelmeyer TD, Cairns FJ. Accidental drowning in Auckland children. *NZ Med J* 1985; **98**: 579–82.
7 Pitt RW, Balanda KP. Childhood drowning and near drowning in Brisbane: the contribution of domestic pools. *Med J Aust* 1991; **154**: 661–5.
8 Health Department of Western Australia. *Preschool drownings in private swimming pools.* Perth: Health Department of Western Australia, 1988.
9 Wintemute GJ. Childhood drowning and near-drowning in the United States. *Am J Dis Child* 1990; **144**: 663 9.
10 Pitt WR. Increasing incidence of child immersion injury in Brisbane. *Med J Aust* 1986; **144**: 683–5.
11 Pearn J, Nixon J. Prevention of childhood drowning accidents. *Med J Aust* 1977; **1**: 16–18.
12 Present P. *Child drowning study: A report on the epidemiology of drownings in residential pools of children under the age of five.* Washington DC: US Consumer Product Safety Commission, 1987.
13 Quan L, Gore W, Wentz K, Allen J, Novak AH. Ten year study of pediatric drownings and near-drowning in Washington: lessons in injury prevention. *Pediatrics* 1989; **83**: 1035–40.
14 Harris A, Warchivker I, de Klerk N. *A review of proposed legislative changes to preschool child drownings in Western Australia: a final report to the Health Department of Western Australia.* Perth: Western Australia, January 1991.
15 Moore M. Many owners may not have to fence pool, says Premier. *Sydney Morning Herald* 1991 September 6.
16 Cook D. Govt made mistakes with pool fencing law, says Metherall. *Sydney Morning Herald* 1991 Sept 5; 3.

17 Elkington J, Carey V, Fowler D. Public perceptions of the New South Wales pool fencing legislation. *Health Promotion J Aust* 1992; **2**: 34–7.

18 Conway R. *The great Australian stupor: an interpretation of the Australian way of life*. Melbourne: Sun Books, 1971.

19 Nixon JW, Pearn JH, Wells R. Child safety and the public media. An analysis from the Brisbane Drowning Study. *Aust Paediatr J* 1980; **16**: 166–8.

20 Pool Fencing Review Committee. *Minority Report of Swimming Pools Fencing Legislation Review. Report to the Minister for Local Government and Co-operatives, New South Wales Government*. Sydney: NSW Parliament, 1992.

21 Steketee M, Coultan M. Court decision may have Greiner biting his bullets. *Sydney Morning Herald* 1991 Dec 11; 4.

22 Garcia LM. Tobacco: Greiner caves in on bans. *Sydney Morning Herald* 1991 Nov 20; 1.

23 Macken L. Gays join Nile by backing 'anti-fags' bill. *Sydney Morning Herald* 1991 Nov 9; 9.

24 Wilkes GA. *A dictionary of Australian colloquialisms*. Sydney: Sydney University Press, 1985: 453–4.

25 Chapman S. On the limitations of econometric analysis in cigarette advertising studies. *Br J Addiction* 1989; **84**: 1267–77.

26 Williams D. Winfield worth more than $8 million to League. *Sydney Morning Herald* 1991 Nov 19; 3.

27 Taylor P. *The smoke ring: the politics of tobacco*. London: Bodley Head, 1985.

28 Deegan L, Thorpe D. RL bosses challenge Carr over smoke bill. *Sunday Telegraph* 1991 Nov 17.

II: A–Z of public health advocacy

5: A–Z of public health advocacy

SIMON CHAPMAN

Michael Pertschuk, a director of the Advocacy Institute in Washington DC, says, "Media advocacy requires art, imagination, and creativity; any effort to reduce it to a series of rigid and prescribed steps is doomed to mediocrity or failure. But practitioners tend to agree on the soundness of certain basic operating principles or practices." This statement summarises well the scope, spirit and intent of this section of the book. It has been my aim to present a comprehensive selection of what most experienced public health advocates would regard as core and commonly encountered strategies, tactics and general guiding principles that should underlie advocacy work.

Introduction

Wherever possible, I have tried to exemplify strategies with at least one case study, which I hope will better enliven the strategy for readers. In most instances, the case studies have been chosen from my own experiences and from those of colleagues working in Australia, the United States, and the United Kingdom. Although I have tried to pick diverse illustrations from the wide field of public health, inevitably the limitations of my own experiences and interests show through. There are plenty of illustrations from the areas of tobacco and gun control, my two main working areas. I have tried hard, however, to detach myself from any content-bound orientation and to address principles of advocacy practice that I hope will be meaningful to public health advocates working in a very wide range of problem areas.

One of the most challenging tasks of teaching in this area is how to make students comfortable with the notion that a two hour session on, say, "dealing with your opposition" or "interview strategies" can only scrape the surface of the range of possibilities that any public health advocate will encounter. In each course that I have taught, there are students who sit expectantly with a fresh notebook hoping to take down a blueprint for promoting any health issue on to the front page or for blasting any anti-public health group out of the water. These students are often disillusioned to find that, even when very experienced and successful public health advocates come along to describe their work, their accounts frequently include vast tracts of untheorised and on-the-run tactics which have of necessity been developed or adapted to fit new, unique, or changing circumstances. This is very much the reality of the day to day of public health advocacy and one of the more important sections in this part of the book is therefore that dealing with *opportunism*.

None the less, most experienced advocates also know that there is considerable method and planning in their work, and I trust that much of this is captured in the pages that follow. Some of the material that follows has been adapted from my 1983 book, *The Lung Goodbye*.[1] Sections of *Columnists, Editorials, Interview Strategies, Letters to the Editor, Media Etiquette, Op-Ed Page Access, Reporters and Journalists*, and *Targeting or Narrowcasting* have been borrowed and adapted from two publications from the Washington DC Advocacy Institute[2 3] with their kind permission.

Not losing sight of the big picture

Before I begin to consider specific strategies, it is important to place advocacy in the wider perspective of the goals it is designed to serve. It is critical that anyone engaging in public health advocacy is clear about the overall public health aims and objectives of the advocacy work in which they are engaged: of the so called "big picture". Failure to understand and constantly reflect on these objectives can cause people to embark on strategies that consume much unproductive energy and, at the end of the day, contribute little to advancing the real public health goals with which advocates should be finally concerned. Advocacy is a *strategy* within public health and, like the adoption of any strategy, decisions about advocacy should result from a disciplined analysis of the problem being addressed. Advocacy should not be seen as an end in itself. Failure to understand this can lead to situations where advocacy objectives override the public health objectives that they were originally designed to meet.

The Advocacy Institute in Washington DC advises:

From the beginning, you should have a good idea of what your media advocacy strategies are trying to accomplish. Review those goals as your messages develop into the framing stages: Are your goals still being met by the way you have framed your issue? Are the goals still appropriate? Finally, when the message has been spread and the results can be seen, take time to evaluate the process you went through. Did anything go wrong, and, if so, how can you frame your message differently the next time? What worked especially well? *Throughout the goals and message process, always keep in mind media advocacy's ultimate aim: to use media to advance your group's public policy goals* [my emphasis].[2]

The main strategies of public health advocacy—media advocacy, political lobbying, community development, and consumer participation in government decision making—can each exert a mesmerising effect on advocates and blind them to the real goals and objectives that these strategies are intended to address. In the case of media advocacy, perhaps the most common confusion of objectives with strategy lies with the mistaking of mere *coverage* in the media with the *purpose* of being covered in the media. The phenomenon of "column inches envy" is widely encountered in the advocacy arena, with many being impressed by the volume of coverage certain issues or spokespeople attract when the far more important issue is whether this volume actually advances the cause that it allegedly is designed to serve.

With most issues, for example, the media have a very short attention span. They may think your issue is fine and newsworthy and give it an avalanche of prominent coverage, lulling you into the belief that you have done all the right things,

131

satisfied the news values and so on. But as we illustrated in the case study on a week of Australian television news in Chapter 3, a mere two or three days later, there will be not a trace of the story in the media: the media will have "consumed" your issue to its satisfaction and moved on to other issues in the never-ending chase for what the very word "news" implies—newness and difference.

A good reminder of this was an interview conducted in the wake of an horrific gun massacre in Australia in 1992. The nation's highest rating current affairs television programme, Channel 9's *A Current Affair*, organised an interview with the mother of a young woman who had been killed in an earlier episode of gun violence. When asked what she would like to see happen regarding gun control, the mother replied that this latest massacre would cause about two days of widespread display of public outcry throughout the media, but then the issue would quietly disappear as she had seen it do several times in response to other massacres since her own daughter's death.

The point to be made here is that providing a sumptuous feast to feed the media's appetite for commentary, perspective, and "angles" on any particular massacre or incident should *not* be seen as the main objective of public health advocacy on gun control. Merely playing out an acclaimed role of outraged expert or anguished community voice against the "evil empire" of the gun lobby may make good television, but may do relatively little to advance gun control tangibly. The objective should be to harness this media appetite in the service of objectives that will lead to reduced gun violence in the community. The power of the media in capturing a nation's attention about an issue should be exploited in the strategic service of objectives such as transforming public concern into public pressure, causing political decision makers to move closer to introducing legislation or laying the foundations that will establish an enduring structure or movement which will assist these processes in the future.

Initial media access can be followed up by new angles on yesterday's story. In the case of the gun massacre, a challenge to all political parties to forget political differences and take a bi-partisan approach to stemming gun violence could lead to interviews with different political leaders and possibly the beginnings of the proposal suggested. Claims made by the gun lobby during their media time can be raked over for their potential to set hares running in new directions that will enhance your media objective in the short term: to contribute to a *sustained* campaign against the gun lobby's interests which, in turn, will, it is to be hoped, translate into increasing public support and political resolve for gun control.

Intrusive ideological baggage

Other common confusions of strategy with objectives result from the intrusion of sacrosanct ideological or professional baggage, often unrelated to the public health objectives in question, which overtake a clear vision of the public health objectives originally being pursued. A good example of this can be seen in the polarisation that often occurs in public health circles over the "top down/bottom up" debate.

Proponents of the bottom up school are convinced that community involvement is absolutely fundamental to the achievement of virtually any public health goal.[4] This conviction arises for them because they do not conceive of community involvement as a strategy, but as an overriding goal in itself. A *developed* community, characterised by an abundance of citizens with a sense of their own power to effect changes within their own community ("empowerment"), is seen as an almost necessary condition to a healthy community. The bottom up school is deeply suspicious of any public health initiative being (as they tend to describe it) "imposed" on populations and tend to equate public indifference to particular health issues as meaning that such health issues are by definition unimportant. To the bottom up proponents, the priority public health problems for a community are those nominated by the community. Uncritically embracing this definition of priorities can leave neglected an embarrassingly large array of often major public health issues which, while failing to animate the public, none the less can have profound consequences for their health status.

Bottom up proponents flirting with notions of public health advocacy will often insist that the best and most efficient ways of encouraging debate and participation about public health policy and legislation are to do it through existing consumer and community networks rather than through the media (sometimes condemned as a classic top down, alienating strategy). Even in the face of an avalanche of evidence that shows that the media are consistently named as the vehicles where most people get most of their knowledge and notions about health issues (*see* Chapter 2), these people insist that discussion of public health issues at the local level, and face to face, is somehow a more legitimate context in which to progress these issues.

A considered analysis of each public health problem will allow the wisdom of such doctrinaire claims to be explored. Such analysis will show that the bottom up "community networks" approach to be appropriate and vital in some instances but inefficient or inappropriate in others. There are many public health problems where community interest in actively taking organised steps to address particular health problems is low and likely to remain so for quite understandable reasons. In my experience, these problems tend to be those that are popularly (and superficially) defined as being problems of unhealthy "lifestyles". There will be very few communities, for example, who will see obvious sense in banding together to help reduce the hypertension rate, the prevalence of sexually transmitted diseases, the incidence of melanoma or teenage smoking. Active "community" interest in lowering such problems will be mostly near enough to zero, even though aggregated individual interest in such issues may well be encouragingly high.

While individuals may thirst for information about how to reduce their personal risk of skin cancer, and be supportive in generally passive ways of legislative moves to remove taxes from skin protection products and hats, it is highly unlikely that hordes of community representatives will regard skin cancer prevention as a health issue sufficiently alarming to warrant significant personal involvement in such top down preventive strategies. If it is agreed that such strategies are vital in a disease reduction programme, it will be far more efficient for cancer control advocates to lobby for their introduction largely independent of community development work. Much time and effort can be wasted in pretending that all public health issues should be addressed using the same principles.

On the other hand, there are many public health problems where local involvement of residents and consumers occurs with a passion. Local street violence, dangerous street crossings, the siting of toxic waste dumps, factories belching smoke into residential areas, lack of after-school care facilities for the children of working parents, poorly maintained pavements, noise pollution and many other "here and now" issues can be very different matters in terms of the interest and commitment of community residents. In such cases, the initial concern about the public health problem will probably have arisen in a local community who will very much "own" it because of its lived, here and now consequences for them.

The top down or "done to" approach is frequently depicted as heinous and Stalinist, whereas "done with" approaches are seen as politically correct and mandatory. This dichotomy is far too simplistic: there are many examples where top down/done to/ upstream strategies in health promotion (so-called passive prevention strategies), initiated by non-consulting health professionals, have been greeted warmly by the public and shown to have benefited public health in important ways.

Random breath testing, comprehensive food labelling, Papanicolaou smears, mandatory bicycle crash helmets and vehicle seat belts, fluoridated water supply, taxes on cigarettes and alcohol, vehicle safety checks and standards . . . this list could go on. All these are hardly popular in the sense that they cause people to take to the streets, many involve things being "done to" people, many have been introduced with next to no involvement or loud expression of interest by consumers, yet many of them are the success stories of modern public health.

In summary then, the first and most critical step in any public health initiative is to conduct an exhaustive problem analysis and then to match the findings of that analysis with appropriate strategies. The role and appropriateness of advocacy strategies will then be apparent and better able to be disciplined by reference to specific objectives that the problem analysis has revealed.

On the next page the issues, tips and detailed discussion of advocacy strategies that form the practical part of this book begin. These are in alphabetical order.

Accuracy

A recent survey of first authors of scientific papers appearing in the *New England Journal of Medicine* found that only 3% of the authors believed that the press coverage their articles had received had been "inaccurate". Importantly, most felt positive about the role of the media in reporting medical and health issues to the public.[5] Despite such studies, many health workers who are wary of dealing with the media cite past experiences of "inaccuracy" in reporting as their main concern. Often, such statements reflect a wholesale misunderstanding of the nature of news reporting: often there is an unreasonable expectation that a newspaper report should be almost like a truncated version of a scientific paper, replete with the same emphases and detached language that are conventional in scientific reports. As we noted in Chapter 2, in the eyes of the media, the big "news" in your study may be perceived quite differently from the emphasis that you as an author would want to see stressed. Such differences in interest or emphasis can create tensions that are not easily resolved. If you are concerned that you might be misquoted or that the issue under discussion runs a high risk of being reported in a technically incorrect or misleading way, it is perfectly sensible to ask a press journalist if he or she might fax you the copy before it goes to press. Do this in a spirit of cooperation and friendliness, not in obvious mistrust. The journalist will also be concerned that his or her report is accurate, because glaring inaccuracies that attract corrections or retractions can make journalists look unprofessional (*see also* Media etiquette).

When you get the draft text of the article, it is imperative that you respect the journalist's need to observe any deadlines that they have specified and get any corrections back to them quickly. If the journalist has put a critical or unkind interpretation or slant on your issue, but has not transgressed any matters of accuracy, you will not be in the same position to offer corrections as when there are simple matters of factual error in the report. Remember that the journalist has not extended the courtesy of allowing you to check the report in order that you might engage them in debate about contentious issues.

Acronyms

If you are forming a public health advocacy group, you will need to give it a name. Journalists generally cannot cope with a negative answer to the question, "Whom do you represent?" The name of your group does not have to be acronymic, but acronymic names for advocacy groups can be catchy and useful in capturing the interest of journalists and the public. An acronym should ideally be a real word or a play on a word that is somehow apposite to, or suggestive of, the issue that a group is addressing, or the actions they are intending to perform (see examples below). Acronyms that spell words that do not exist —for example, IBFAN: International Baby Food Action Network —or allude to nothing meaningful require people not only to inquire about what the letters in the words stand for, but also to remember a vocabulary of new names that do not trigger apposite associations.

When should an acronymic name be used? Most groups who decide to use acronyms tend to be fringe groups with confrontational agendas, which operate outside the more established non-government organisations (NGOs). Establishment NGOs have a more sober, serious sense of themselves often bound up with needing to appeal to the broad and conservative public for donations and bequests.[6] Acronyms, especially those that are strident or irreverent, do not sit well with such bodies. This can often mean that establishment organisations will be reluctant to be seen to associate with acronymic groups, even when they are working towards the same cause. The conservative groups fear that association with radical groups may be perceived by the public as meaning that they share all aspects of the radical groups' agenda and strategies. That they often do not goes a long way to explaining why radical groups sometimes decide to form (see Radicalism).

Acronymic names have historically connoted radicalism, irreverence, and mocking, a "gloves-off" approach to campaigning, and a more ephemeral existence for the group. They are seldom listed in a telephone directory, for example. Such objectives and the strategies that are consistent with them often have an important role in public health advocacy. The decision, therefore, to name your group with an acronym should consider whether this is the sort of profile and set of expectations you wish to foster.

Examples of reader friendly acronyms are:

- ACT UP (AIDS Coalition to Unleash Power)
- AGHAST (Action Groups to Halt Advertising and Sponsorship of Tobacco)
- ASH (Action on Smoking and Health)
- BUGA UP (Billboard Utilising Graffitists Against Unhealthy Promotions)
- DOC (Doctors Ought to Care)
- MADD (Mothers Against Drunk Drivers)
- MOP UP (Movement Opposed to the Promotion of Unhealthy Products)
- TREES (Those Resisting Environmental Effluent from Smoking).

Advertising in advocacy

Advocacy advertising[7] is the purchasing of space or broadcast time to have your issue publicised in a fully controlled, unedited way. Because the advertiser controls the text, script and layout, nothing needs to be left to chance that journalists will put the desired inflection on your message. Advertising is a means of guaranteeing that a message you wish to have publicised or broadcast will be run in exactly the way, with exactly the wording and illustrations or imagery that you want. Advertising costs money, however, with the rule of thumb being that the greater the size of the audience or readership, the greater the cost. This means that on national issues, when you want to achieve mass attention, or whenever your goal is to have other media run stories on your advertising, huge costs will often be involved. Unless your agency is well funded or you have a philanthropic benefactor, such advertising will generally be out of reach and you will need to rely on newsmaking and publicity to get your messages out. This is the situation of the overwhelming majority of advocacy groups working in the public health field.

There are hundreds of books, courses, consultants and, of course, advertising agencies themselves that offer advice on how to achieve optimal results through advertising. Such advice lies beyond the scope of this book, save for mention of one potentially inexpensive way that poorly funded advocacy groups can use this medium.

Signature "petition" advertising

Statements and "open letters" (*see* Open letters) to politicians, regulatory authorities, or industries can be published as paid advertisements with a long list of signatories below the text of the statement or letter (see figure 1). The idea is to share the cost of the advertisement by having each signatory contribute. Many individuals and agencies like to see their name in print and, moreover, will feel doubly concerned about their name being absent from a long published list of prominent people or peers supporting an issue with which they would want to be identified. If you have a network of agencies that support your cause, the text of the letter should be circulated with a request that those wishing to sign should fax or phone their approval to the organisers. Payment should quickly follow as most newspapers will insist on prepayment for large advertisements placed by groups that do not have regular advertising accounts.

Once you know the price of the size and placement of advertisement you require, you will be able to calculate how many signatories you will need if you are to request contributions that are within the means of your supporters. When a minimum number of signatories has been gathered, you can then decide on whether to gather more and make the exercise into a fund raising venture.

If your list of signatories includes celebrities (*see* Celebrities), ask them if they can suggest other celebrities who are likely to sign. Celebrities tend to know and associate with other celebrities and may have access to their unlisted phone numbers, which will save you a lot of time. Celebrity and authority signatures on the advertisement will add to its news value.

The advertisement may well become newsworthy in itself (*see* Media cannibalism) and the media may want to interview some signatories on why they signed and so on. By going public, your signatories must accept some responsibility for their views, but it is likely that some people who sign will not have up to date and accurate information and may become a liability to the cause if they are interviewed without being properly briefed. Where possible, you should follow up any agreement to sign with information kits or fact sheets, and offer to assist with briefings if any media follow up occurs.

139

Decriminalisation of marijuana

— a call for action!

We, the undersigned, call on the leaders of Australia to make a decisive choice in favour of the better of two (2) alternatives as to what the law should do relating to Marijuana. We call upon Governments in this country to decriminalise the use of Marijuana forthwith. The community can no longer continue the existing policy of prohibition, a proven failure. Governments must opt positively for decriminalisation.

The war to stamp out personal use of Marijuana has failed, the war has been lost, respect for the law is not universal and when there is not a respect for the law, the law is held in contempt by a percentage of the community. Throughout the community enlightened opinion has been moving apace towards recognition of the fact that in terms of the balance of weights, the arguments in favour of decriminalisation dramatically outweigh those supportive of self defeating perpetuation of the prevailing prohibition policy, a policy which is not succeeding.

As with alcohol in the United States 3 generations ago, prohibition has been an economic boom beyond calculation to the worst criminal elements in the population who have profited from the illegality of Marijuana to the tune of millions and millions of dollars. There is not sufficiently strong public will to enforce the ban. The social cost of Marijuana abuse is infinitesimal compared with similar costs associated with alcohol and tobacco abuse.

We, the undersigned, do not suggest that severe overuse of Marijuana is not harmful. We do, however, say quite clearly that the present policy has not the respect of the community and needs review, needs new impetus and needs the law makers to act to ensure that there is respect for the law.

MR. PHILLIP ADAMS A.O.
THE ADDICTION STUDIES UNIT, SCHOOL OF PSYCHOLOGY, CURTIN UNIVERSITY
PROF. PETER & MRS. J BAUME A.O.
MR DON BAXTER, AIDS COUNCIL OF AUSTRALIA
MR DAVID BENNETT, Q.C.
MR BERNARD D. BRASSIL, B.A. LL.B. SOLICITOR
MR KEN BUCKLEY
PROF. PETER BROOKS M.S. B.S. M.D.
THE HONOURABLE MEREDITH BURGMANN, M.L.C.
DR SIMON CHAPMAN
DR ALEX COHEN
MR G.B. CHESHER
PROF. DONALD J. CHISHOLM M.B. B.S.
MR PETER CLEELAND, CHAIRPERSON OF THE JOINT PARLIAMENTARY COMMITTEE ON THE NATIONAL CRIME AUTHORITY
MISS SHARRON CREWS, B.A. LL.B.
MS PHYLL DANCE
DR MICHAEL DAWSON, UTS UNIVERSITY
DR MICHAEL DAWSON,
PROFESSOR RICHARD DAY M.B. B.S. M.D.
MR B.H.K. DONOVAN Q.C.
DR ERNEST DRUCKER, PH.D.
DRUG REFERRAL INFORMATION CENTRE

DR JOHN ELLARD A.M.
THE HONOURABLE RUSSELL FOX, A.C. Q.C.
IAN S. FRASER, ASSOCIATE PROFESSOR OF OBSTETRICS AND GYNAECOLOGY UNIVERSITY OF SYDNEY
THE HONOURABLE A.T. GIETZELT, A.O.
MR PETER GROGAN, PRESIDENT OF AIDS COUNCIL OF NEW SOUTH WALES
MS LEONE HEALY
THE HONOURABLE RICHARD JONES, M.L.C.
EMERIT. PROF. P. KARMEL, A.C.
MS JOAN S. KERSEY
MR PHILIP KING LLB
MR CRAIG KNOWLES, M.P.
MR JOHN MARSDEN LL.M.
MR IAN MATHEWS, A.M.
MS ALLANAH MacTIERNAN B.A., B. JURIS. LL.B. M.L.C., J.P. M.P.
THE HONOURABLE J.R. McCLELLAND B.A. LL.B.
THE HONOURABLE MS JEAN McLEAN, M.L.C.
MS M.E. McNISH
MR GRAEME P. MONTEITH
MR MICHAEL MOORE, M.P.
DR STEPHEN MUGFORD
MR STEPHEN MURPHY, B.E. (CHEM) (HONS).
MR WILLIAM O'BRIEN, B. JURIS. LL.B.

THE HONOURABLE PAUL O'GRADY M.P.
MR W.G. PETERSEN
SENATOR MARGARET REYNOLDS
PROFESSOR BILL SAUNDERS
MR JIM SNOW, M.H.R. MEMBER FOR EDEN-MONARO
MS ELIZABETH SKINNER, DRUG REFERRAL INFORMATION CENTRE
SENATOR SID SPINDLER, AUSTRALIAN DEMOCRATS, SENATOR FOR VICTORIA
THE HONOURABLE ANN SYMONDS, M.L.C.
MR PETER TREBILCO
DR I. VAN BEEK, DIRECTOR, KIRKETON ROAD CENTRE
MS TINA VAN RAAY, SECRETARY AUSTRALIAN PARLIAMENTARY GROUP ON DRUG LAW REFORM
M. WALTON AND ROBERT PULLAN
MRS MARION WATSON
PROF. IAN WEBSTER, M.D.B.S.
DR EDITH WEISBERG
DR PAUL WILSON, DEAN OF HUMANITIES BOND UNIVERSITY
ALEX & JO WODAK
MR KIM YEADON M.P.
MR PETER YELDHAM. O.A.M.
NSW YOUNG LAWYERS

Figure 1: Prominent Australians speak out in a paid advertisement advocating drug law reform.

Case study: analogies

In the late 1980s the Australian Consumers' Association (ACA) was lobbying to safeguard and improve grocery product labelling in the face of a sustained food industry campaign to deregulate labelling standards. The food industry framed their position in terms of survey data which showed that many consumers do not read food labels and by arguing that the labelling requirements included overly restrictive definitions of ingredients that inhibited innovation and product development, thus being against the interest of consumers. The ACA countered with the standard arguments about people with allergies and food intolerances being placed in danger by the deregulatory proposals. This line appeared somewhat stale to journalists, however, and was easily countered by statements from the industry that the deregulatory directions being proposed would safeguard the preservation of relevant labelling in such cases.

ACA then produced an inspired analogy-based reframing when it held a press conference to make the point that labelling on pet food was more comprehensive and comprehensible than that on grocery items for human consumption. Its theme, that Fido the dog (who couldn't read) was already provided with a level of information about his doggie dinner that was being denied to his owners about their food, provided a powerful illustration of the folly of the industry's position. The industry campaign quickly ran out of steam.

Analogies, metaphors, and similes

The use of analogy, metaphor, and simile can be powerful ways of efficiently and memorably translating your issue into concepts and comparisons that are likely to mean more to people. A voluntary, unenforced code on passive smoking in the workplace could be described as being "as useless as an ashtray on a motorbike." When the British Prime Minister Margaret Thatcher

Case study: analogies

In 1993, pressure from motoring lobbies in New South Wales caused the police to announce a change in policy about the location of speed cameras. Since their introduction, the cameras had been hidden so that speeding motorists could not see them ahead and slow down only until they had passed the cameras. There was widespread and vocal public support for bringing the cameras out into the open, with most of this support being framed in terms of the cameras being a "revenue raising exercise" by a mismanaged government rather than an important road injury reduction strategy. The reframing was proving astonishingly powerful, capturing public cynicism about government policy. In response, the Public Health Association put out the following press release in which the two italicised analogies were emphasised in the many interviews that resulted.

FOR IMMEDIATE RELEASE 7 JUNE 1993

The Public Health Association has questioned the decision by the NSW police to stop the practice of hiding speed cameras and instead locate them only where they can be clearly seen by motorists.

The Association believes the decision reflects an over-sensitivity to community complaints from those who have been caught speeding red-handed and that the police seem to have lost the plot about the deterrence of speeding.

Dr Simon Chapman, National Vice-President of the Association said it was astonishing that police seemed to have lost sight of the very reason for hidden speed cameras. "Any street-wise yahoo intent on speeding will simply slow down in areas known to have speed cameras and carry on endangering life wherever else they please. *This decision makes as much sense as having shop detectives wear uniforms or customs agents announcing which flights they will search for drugs.*"

"*To argue that hidden cameras should be condemned because they raise revenue is like arguing that catching burglars is wrong because it creates employment for prison officers.* The whole point is that hidden speed cameras are designed to make drivers slow down by raising concern that a camera could be around the next bend."

142

Case study: analogies

During a protracted debate over reforming health warnings on Australian cigarette packs, Dr Brendon Nelson (president of the Australian Medical Association) argued that rat poison sold in shops carried the explicit label that it "killed rats and mice" whereas tobacco pack warnings did not carry wording that the product could kill users despite 20 000 Australians annually dying from tobacco use (figure 2).

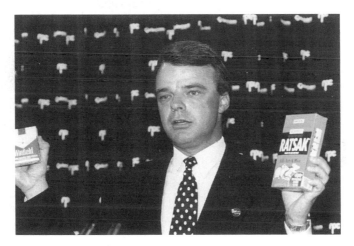

Figure 2: Dr Brendon Nelson, Australian Medical Association President, making an apposite point on packet labelling.

awarded an export award to a tobacco company, David Simpson, then director of Britain's Action on Smoking and Health, described the award as being "like a rabid dog winning Cruft's Dog Show." The appointment of a representative of your opposition to a role where their vested interests are likely to be safeguarded or promoted can evoke the time honoured "it's like putting Dracula in charge of the blood bank."

Anniversaries

Many public health issues have significant events as mileposts, such as catastrophes—for example, gun massacres, notorious chemical spills, and fires, deaths of significant or famous people who died from particular diseases or who were leaders in your field, the publication of expert reports or inquiries, and government decisions or back-offs. Journalists will sometimes flag such events in their diaries and on the anniversaries of such events, will seek to present "revisit" stories. These typically examine progress, ask "Has anything been done?" questions, explore whether the same problems are still happening, review progress on the promises made at the time by authorities and politicians, and so on.

Advocates know about these milestones more than any others in the community, but too seldom plan to exploit them, opting rather simply to react to approaches from those journalists who take the initiative. More often, anniversaries which could give rise to large and positive media coverage are completely overlooked. Here are some actions that you should take.

- Note all significant anniversaries on planning charts and calendars; enter them into electronic diaries or computers so that they are flagged automatically for you some weeks before they arrive.
- Contact journalists weeks before these anniversaries, reminding them and suggesting angles that they may wish to pursue.
- Contact and brief appropriate spokespeople who could give expert or personal commentary on the event or issue.
- Undertake any creative calculations that relate to the passage of time since the anniversary (for example, the number of road deaths on an accident prone stretch of road since a government refused to act on a proposed re-routing—a "we warned you" story; number of children drowned in domestic pools since failure of campaign to make surround fences compulsory).
- Consider whether there is any scope for sending a very public anniversary present to friends or foes of public health.
- Plan and organise any media events or stunts that might break through media indifference to the anniversary.

Be there! The first rule of advocacy

There are critical political decision making forums in every society, whether these be parliamentary, religious, local governmental, or even nepotistic. Public health advocates need to understand the way these operate. Who is known to have influence with a targeted health minister or politician? With their political peers? With their marginal seat colleagues? With members of their families? With particular friends or friends of family members? With their church leaders? With someone in their tennis groups or ski lodge? Where is the real business of a political party forged? This sort of information needs to be gathered and exploited through all the other principles of opportunism, networking, framing, and so on discussed in this section of the book.

The elementary principle of "being there" needs translation into the multitude of opportunities that can be important in public health advocacy. If, for example, you work in an institution such as a large hospital or university, and know that certain administrative or planning committees are where potential public health relevant decisions could be taken, try and get yourself or a trusted representative appointed to that committee. If you succeed, this may involve many hours of attending to matters that are wholly distant from public health matters—valuable time that you might consider wasted. If, however, your membership of the committee leads to the passage of important policies that would be unlikely to have been raised or supported in your absence, what more is there to say?

Personal friendships with key decision makers can also be critical avenues of influence. In leaked tobacco industry debriefing material obtained by the American tobacco control advocacy group, DOC (Doctors Ought to Care), there is a plain speaking example of how this can work. Referring to the defeat of a tobacco tax in Arizona, the document says "[an industry lobbyist] has done a great job with his first session as our lobbyist. He is best friends with the Speaker and used major personal clout to kill our cigarette tax."[8]

Bluff

In advocacy, as in poker, bluff can be an important tactic that can cause your opponents to act unwisely. Saul Alinsky wrote, "Power is not only what you have but what the enemy thinks you have."[9] This principle can have special meaning to small, unfunded community groups engaged in public health advocacy against foes who are formidably powerful. Bluff in advocacy work can mean anything from cultivating a deliberate ambiguity about the size of your group to allusions about the extent of your contacts within your opponents' ranks (*see* Infiltration). Your opponents may well be adept bluffers as well. So again, as in poker, calling the bluff of your opponents in advocacy can sometimes precipitate ill advised moves by them that may advantage your cause.

Boycotts

The call for the boycott of a service, institution, or product, formidable as it can sound, is probably the most overused and ineffective "strategy" in public health advocacy. This is because there is a world of difference between simply *calling* for a boycott and successfully *organising* a boycott. And mostly, boycotts are simply called for, rather than organised in a sustained way that enables them to achieve their intended objectives. It is not difficult to recall many examples of outraged health workers or consumers venting their spleens and calling for all concerned people to boycott products made by a company that has in some way offended or exploited. But there are few examples of boycotts that have actually worked, hurting their targets and causing changes to occur in the factors that inspired the boycott.

The call for a boycott carries with it the powerful subtext that the product or service in question is in some way morally reprehensible. Consequently, a highly publicised call for a boycott may lend a degree of negative publicity to the object of the boycott. But recalling the discussion in Chapter 3 of the transitory, ephemeral nature of news, a mere call for a boycott will probably gain publicity once or twice, whereas the boycott process and its results will be a different matter. In summary then, do not abuse the potential power of a boycott by merely hurling the word into the media ether if you have not given extensive commitment to following through with the threat.

Successful boycotts are easiest to organise at a local level, where loss of trade or customers by, for example, a cinema complex that refuses to install access ramps for patrons in wheelchairs or a hospital canteen that insists on stocking cigarettes can be realistically organised. It should not need to be said that a boycott in such circumstances should be a last resort, following representations to the offending outlet, then publicity about its inaction, and perhaps other lobbying strategies such as customer petitions and picketing.

Boycotts of nationally or internationally available products —for example, the international Nestlé product boycott[10]—are a quite different matter. These can take years of careful planning and organisation.

Boycotts by celebrities

Celebrities such as athletes or performers can themselves boycott products or opportunities to compete or perform in ways that often focus the media on their reasons for doing so.

Case study: boycotts

Many sports have annual "best player" awards donated by tobacco companies. The major rugby league competition in Sydney has one such award, the Rothmans Medal, which attracts great following in the media. The award is determined by secret voting of a panel and there is immense speculation about who will win the award in the preceding weeks. In 1982, on the day before the final judging, I issued a press release calling on whoever won the medal to refuse to accept it as a gesture towards acknowledging the example they would set to children. The release generated large stories about the issue in several papers and was raised several times by the television commentators during the programme. The winner turned out to be an employee of Rothmans itself.

When you know an event such as a tournament, festival, or concert is approaching which is sponsored by your opposition, try to contact all players known to be competing in the tournament, pointing out how their participation will be used to promote your opposition's product or values. Point out how inconsistent this is with the responsibility to promote health that you are sure the player subscribes to, and that the player should be aware that a lot of adverse publicity will be stirred up by your movement at the time of the event.

Some of these people may be strongly supportive of your suggestion but unwilling to withdraw from the event. They may none the less be willing to make some public statement to the effect that the system virtually necessitates their competing in such events because international sporting administration declares (for example) that tobacco sponsored events are major tournaments that have bearing on players' world rankings. If a player speaks out about being thus compromised, a powerful subtext of unfairness will surround the event in the eyes of the public.

There need not be massive or even majority support within a sport or a field of the arts for boycotts or criticism to work in sending anti-public health sponsors skulking away. In Britain in 1984, Paul Eddington and Warren Mitchell were two leading actors who gave public support to Artists Against Smoking Sponsorship. Eddington, with his vast experience in the theatre, claimed that sponsors were "like shy horses" who needed every encouragement to back events and could be put off by the slightest discouragement.

Bureaucratic constraints

Many people working in public health are employed by government departments or agencies, or by NGOs with conservative political agendas. Bureaucrats are often frustrated by the political impasses or inertia under which they are obliged to work. Often they will report a real conflict between their professional assessment of what should be done to further stated government policy and their growing knowledge that certain important actions are "politically unacceptable" in the wider context of government, perhaps conflicting with other portfolios such as agriculture, labour, and industry. Government, for example, may be underfunding public health campaigns or refusing to implement policy or legislation that is vital to a public health objective. Such situations can create tensions and conflict between the professional views of those ostensibly employed by government to (say) reduce the road toll or the availability of unsafe goods, and the sense of duty that they are supposed to feel towards the policies of the government that employs them. Their own ideals become compromised and their roles are reduced to appearing to protect politicians' careers. This frustration can often breed a willingness to help outsiders by precipitating courses of action that they themselves cannot be seen to participate in, but which, once placed on the government agenda, they may be able to manipulate to advantage.

The classic ways of bureaucrats helping are by leaking documents and by forewarning of events, meetings, and impending announcements, thus enabling anticipatory action by public health groups in the community. Bureaucrats will be the best judge of what is potentially useful and of their own security in leaking particular pieces of information. They may be able to suggest prudent times for writing certain letters, or to provide valuable background information that might assist the content and timing of your submissions to politicians.

One view of government bureaucracy is that the duty of those working in it is to provide unquestioning support for the policies of the government of the day. If the government is going soft on a polluting industry, the duty of an environmental health bureaucrat, according to this view, is not to take any actions that might provoke a change in government policy or practice. Rather, the bureaucrat is expected to offer or suppress advice and information in ways that will best serve the government policy of the day. We are not writing this book for those who subscribe to this view, but rather for public health workers (including government bureaucrats) dedicated to improving public health outcomes. This section offers some advice about how to circumvent such bureaucratic constraints and oil the wheels of public health advocacy from inside government or conservative organisations.

A note of caution: it is wise to be on guard about your relationship with bureaucrats. Double-bind situations can arise

149

where your independence can be severely compromised through "past favours owed". In a situation of conflicting wishes—of bureaucrats wanting to tone you down for fear that you will embarrass their department over inactivity or such like—awkward decisions must sometimes be made.

Depressed economic environments are known to reduce the road toll because people drive less when money is scarce and public transport is used more.[11] In the lead up to the 1993 Australian federal election, the conservative (Liberal) opposition party made the electorally popular promise that they would dramatically reduce the price of fuel by eliminating sales taxes on petroleum. Government road safety officers knew that this electoral gimmick would mean many extra lives would be lost on the roads, yet those who worked in states governed by Liberal governments were uniformly silent in speaking out against the proposed cuts in petrol tax. The Liberal opposition was widely tipped to win the forthcoming election and many road safety officials feared that to speak out against a prominent election promise would bring down the wrath of their state Liberal government employers who would see such criticism as overtly political (which, unavoidably, it was).

The issue was eventually raised by a report strategically ordered and then published by the sitting Federal Labor Government,[12] but the dilemma illustrated here is very common, and can present huge problems for government employees or agencies receiving government funding (who fear that criticism of government may turn off the funding tap). The following are some of the more usual ways around such constraints.

Leaks

Leaking is anonymous whistleblowing (*see* Whistleblowers). Leaked documents that "fall off the back of a truck" are a veritable media institution as old as the newspaper scoop itself. Leaked documents are generally headlined as such, lending them a mystery of secretiveness, suggesting cover ups and intriguing divisions within the organisation that is leaking. The subtext of a leak is that there is someone within the leaking agency or committee who wants to share a forbidden secret. And secrets, by their nature, are beguiling. A journalist who receives a leak will often feel more privileged than his or her colleagues for having been selected by the leaker to receive the information. This may translate into a more sympathetic and detailed coverage of the issue involved than would be the case with a routine press release that was sent to all media.

If you are a bureaucrat, it may be that you are in a position to leak information or documents yourself. You may also be able to coax leaks out of particular organisations, industries, or committees. If you are considering issuing a leak yourself, it is obviously wise to think hard about the consequences that may flow both to your issue and to you or your colleagues should the source of the leak be traced. Once you have decided to go ahead, it will generally be important to consider whether you wish potentially to martyr yourself as a whistleblower or how best to cover your tracks and how to give the leaked information the momentum that you might hope for it.

Issues to consider include: are you breaking any law by your proposed leak (if you are, the police may become involved)? How easily might the leak be traced to you or to your colleagues? How many other people have access to the information? Will it be assumed that it is you who has leaked the information? Are there identifying marks on the copy that you will leak that can be traced to you? If you are sending material by fax, is your sender's number going to be printed on the faxed copy (you can usually turn this facility off)?

Community development

Many governments subscribe, at least in their rhetoric, to the principles and philosophies of community development. To the unsuspecting conservative politician or bureaucrat, "community development" can sound like a benign and harmless process where relatively small amounts of money are siphoned into community groups to enable them to do politically innocuous things such as beautify public spaces, advise on community services, and so on. The expectation is that such a process will be good for local electoral "pump priming": locally visible projects will occur and their organisers will probably express their gratitude and provide many photo opportunities for beneficent politicians—all very good for re-election prospects.

In fact, the nature of the problems that need "developing" in communities will often involve conflicts with existing government policies. Consequently, the community development process can often foment groups of citizens who can become key players in the public health advocacy process. There are a great many examples in the contemporary public health scene where the role of consumer advocacy has been absolutely critical to the advancement of public health goals. These are particularly issues where government employees' hands are tied in being unable to criticise, lobby, and generally advocate for health issues where government policy is not in the best interests of health. In such circumstances consumer and community groups quickly become the leading edge of advocacy.

Such groups can usually be relied on by journalists to "shoot from the hip" about public health issues in contrast to the guarded equivocations of establishment agency or government representatives. Independent groups can decide for themselves far more flexibly than their established counterparts not only what should be said and done about public health issues, but the style in which these actions might be executed.

An active climate of consumer advocacy can act as a safeguard against a sycophantic *"Yes Minister"* decision making environment, and can force high profile public consideration of issues which will often be critical of government policy. If policy, programmes, and resource allocations are made by people only mindful of the political acceptability of particular positions, there will be very many instances of the health agenda being emasculated or wholly neglected. The often spectacular achievements of advocacy groups such as ACT UP, ASH, and Greenpeace are illustrative of the power of non-government agencies to influence policy.

If you work for government and anticipate that a political era is approaching in which there will be many conflicts between government policy and public health, try to use the rhetoric of community development or consumer participation as a Trojan horse to ensure that uncompromised, independent voices from the community will be put in place and heard during the lean times that are likely to follow. The same principle applies to allowing academics, traditionally the other main source of independent views, to play an active part in the advocacy process.

Using the seemingly benign rhetoric of community development or sponsoring academically independent assessments, try to set up enduring structures for consultation, funding, and participation in planning, organisation, and evaluation which require community members and academics to be involved.

Fostering such involvement will often be seen by politicians as entirely positive when expressed in the abstract, rather than in specific terms of introducing "loose canons" (sic) into particular policy debates. If you can be astute in establishing and safeguarding such structures, consultation processes, and funding arrangements in ways that make them genuinely open to the community (and not just to "community" political stooges or yea-sayers), then you will find policy forums invigorated with public health perspectives that will often be challenging to conservative government policies.

Celebrities

Celebrities, by definition, are newsworthy. If Margaret Russell (who?) has breast cancer, there is probably no news value in this unless she is receiving some new treatment, has been subjected to some form of negligence or neglect, or fulfils any of the other subtextual criteria illustrated in Chapters 2 and 3. But if Olivia Newton-John, the singer/actress, reveals that she has breast cancer (as was the case in 1992), the media will give immense coverage not only to her condition but also to the issues involved in breast cancer generally. Celebrity illnesses and injuries, or even those of their families, fascinate the media and can provide valuable vehicles for sympathetic coverage of health issues.

In our study of Sydney press reportage of health issues in five months of 1993, of 4019 press reports coded, 8% concerned people who were international or national identities. These included reports on the cause of the deaths of Rudolph Nureyev and Arthur Ashe (AIDS), Audrey Hepburn and Pat Nixon (cancer), illness in Mother Teresa, Olivia Newton-John (breast cancer), and Princess Diana's bulimic eating disorder.

Public health advocates need to plan how to respond to news of a celebrity death or illness. This will require a great deal of sensitivity, particularly if there is any potential for an interpretation to be made that you are in any way "dancing on the grave" or exploiting the misfortune of the celebrity. If the celebrity is still alive, it is critical that you make contact with him or her before making any statement to the media and determine whether the celebrity is likely to be supportive of any comments you may be making. If you intend making comments about the preventability of a disease affecting a celebrity, a subtext that may be problematic is one that says "Celebrity X has lung cancer. Most lung cancer is preventable if people didn't smoke. X smoked and now has lung cancer. Therefore we are suggesting that X has been rather foolish." Although such a subtext will apply to many preventable diseases where discretionary behaviour is involved, it should be avoided.

If the celebrity has died, careful thought should also be given to the way in which you couch your comments on the death. In 1992, a prominent Australian footballer was killed in a car crash. His death was reported all over the front pages of Sydney newspapers and was the leading item on television and radio news. The reports all focused on the widespread grief that the death was causing in the footballer's working class district. He had been a member of a team that had won the premiership the year before and put a huge amount of pride into an economically depressed area.

All media reports on the death avoided any speculation about the cause of the crash, despite the furious sweep of a rumour that the footballer had been drinking heavily in the hours before the crash. Road trauma authorities were well aware of the rumours, which would have been very easy to corroborate, but made no comment. A few days later, his brother made a statement to the media confirming that the footballer had indeed been driving with a high blood alcohol level at the time of the crash. The statement again made front page headlines.

It is interesting to speculate on what public reception would have been given to an exposé of the drink factor, had it been made by someone other than a member of his family. Road trauma authorities apparently weighed the probability of a backlash against their intrusion into the grief of the district against the likelihood that either the footballer's family member or the government coroner would soon announce the inevitable. Their decision to keep silent was probably wise, resulting in the

"Don't drink and drive" message being delivered with an authenticity that they could never have commanded.

Contacting celebrities

Celebrities, in voicing their views on health issues, can also be valuable advocates for public health. Prince Charles, for example, has made many public statements about urban blight and poor planning which have been widely reported and generated debate. The late Zairian guitarist and band leader Franco Luambo Makiadi, who enjoyed a massive following throughout francophone and east Africa spanning 25 years, assisted in AIDS and immunisation campaigning work through his music. Another example is actor Elizabeth Taylor's efforts to publicise AIDS issues. Her "star" attention-drawing quality has ensured high media coverage whenever she seeks it. Advocates can do much better than simply waiting for a celebrity to announce their views on a health issue and then trying to contact them. Hints and clues that a celebrity may be sympathetic to your issue can be gleaned from interviews or reported comments they make on similar areas and so on. If you suspect that a celebrity is on your side, try to contact them and ask them directly if they can help. How can you contact celebrities? It is interesting just how many people know a celebrity, or know someone well who knows a celebrity. Ask around. This may turn up someone who will be in a good position to contact them and get a more favourable outcome. Do you know someone who went to school with the person? Who is a neighbour? Whose child is in the same class as the celebrity's child? Who knows the wife or husband of the celebrity? There are many ways that this can happen.

Failing this, most celebrities have agents who look after their bookings and protect them from the public. A phone call to any of the big management agencies will quickly give you the name and contact details of the agency which handles the celebrity you are after. Working through an agent can sometimes be a disadvantage, because you will be obliged to deal through an intermediary who may be unsympathetic to your issue and will not present it well to the celebrity.

Untrained cannons?

There are also problems associated with using celebrities. It may be that a celebrity agrees with your policies only on a limited basis or in a very superficial way, and that when unleashed before an inquiring media, embarrassing differences may emerge. If you are going to use a celebrity, you must feel entirely comfortable that they are thoroughly briefed about the issue and the likely line of questioning from both supportive and hostile media. Before committing a celebrity to any particular role in your advocacy campaign, it is very wise to develop a good understanding of their strengths and weaknesses and to tailor the role accordingly.

The issue of sincerity is also a problem. Audiences have become accustomed to celebrities giving paid testimonials for all products via advertising. To avoid the suspicion that a celebrity is being paid for their involvement, it is important that he or she is personally committed to the issue and is not simply taking the role to enhance his or her public image. Finally, you should be on guard against the media becoming infatuated with the human interest angle provided by the celebrity if this angle threatens to overwhelm other essential but possibly less "interesting" facets of your campaign.

Chain letters

To most people, chain letters are annoyances we occasionally receive from "get rich quick" schemes. The principle involved, however, can be put to good use in public health advocacy. Chain letters have the potential to deliver many thousands of letters supporting your cause to a particular target, such as a politicians as the following case study illustrates.

Case study: chain letters

In 1986, the Minister for Health in South Australia, Dr John Cornwall, was about to introduce a comprehensive tobacco control Bill into the State parliament. I was working with the Minister and he told me that some of his ministerial colleagues took the view that tobacco control was not an issue that was electorally popular. Further, the tobacco industry was expected to mount its usual lobbying campaign which would involve assisting shopkeepers and those who were currently benefiting from tobacco sponsorships in sport and the arts, to pressure their local politicians on the issue.

Dr Cornwall asked me to think about ways of sending major signals from the community to his parliamentary colleagues. Past efforts to pass tobacco control legislation, he said, had been characterised by vocal support from the expected sources: the medical profession and anti-tobacco lobby groups. Although it was important that these groups continued to be seen to be committed to the proposed legislation, they suffered the political disadvantage of being comparatively small in number and, above all, quite predictable in their support.

The challenge became one of how to mobilise a mass and rapid display of public support from the wider community. One of the major tactics was an attempt to light the fuse of a chain letter. The South Australian Anti Cancer Foundation was obviously supportive of the proposed legislation and had written letters of support to the Health Minister and the Premier, sent deputations of senior specialists and experts to visit the Minister (who needed no persuading), and engaged in considerable media commentary on the proposals. The Foundation had a mailing list of some 6000 people in the State who regularly donated money for cancer research, education, and patient support. I proposed to the Foundation's Director that he should write to each of these 6000 donors, urging them to send a letter of support to the Minister of Health. He agreed.

A letter was sent which explained how important the legislation would be for cancer prevention. It urged each donor to write to the Minister and to copy the letter of request to six friends or colleagues, who thus would in turn be asked to do the same. The letter listed a series of points that each writer might consider making in their letter to the Minister (see Letters to politicians). Urgency was stressed, and a final dateline for the exercise was emphasised. Each writer was urged to add to their letter that "no reply was requested", thus saving the Minister's office from a potentially massive and costly acknowledgement response. Specifying a deadline is very important so as to avoid chain letters continuing well after an advocacy initiative is finished.

The exercise worked extremely well, with some 11 000 personally written letters supporting the Health Minister pouring into his office in the ensuing weeks. These were bundled up into boxes and then stacked on a trolley. During the parliamentary debate, Dr Cornwall had a trolley laden with these apparently spontaneously penned letters wheeled into the parliamentary chamber. In another pile, he bundled the 20 or so letters of complaint he had received from a group of taxi drivers and tobacconists who opposed the Bill. The contrast was complete and dramatically underscored the community support for the Bill.

Columnists

To supplement their editorial pages, newspapers print columns by regular columnists such as social commentators, retired politicians, or celebrities. Some syndicated columnists are published in several papers, large and small. Most papers also have their own columnists who write on a variety of local and national issues.

Developing a relationship with a columnist is similar to developing a relationship with a reporter. You will be better off if you develop long term relationships with the columnists who publish in your local paper. Once they know and trust you, it will be much easier for you to influence what they write.

Start by knowing which columnists publish in your paper. Even if they are nationally syndicated and headquartered elsewhere, if they write about subjects relevant to your area of interest, it is important to make contact with them. Columnists, like all reporters, are always hungry for new ideas and good information. In many ways columnists are more hungry than reporters because they don't have editors telling them what to write and they know that they must produce their column on a regular basis (ordinary journalists can often afford to have slow news days—their bylines will not be missed by readers as much as a columnist).

Know the columnist's style and predilections. Making an inappropriate suggestion for a column will waste your time and that of the columnist. Some, for example, will have no interest in the struggles of a local health care centre. Others will probably not want to hear about your evidence of corruption or ineptitude in the local bureaucracy. If they want a specific type of story idea or information from you, get it to them as soon as possible. A continuing relationship with a columnist is a very valuable resource that should be nurtured. Columnists, because of their prominence, will want *exclusives* even more than reporters.

Crank letters (or how to put your opposition's worst foot forward)

Occasionally you will be handed an opportunity to choose your opponent in a debate, or someone who will respond to your comments or initiatives. A journalist may ask, "Is there anyone you can think of [from your opposition] whom I could contact to comment on your statement?" On such occasions, consider the value of promoting the worst example of your opposition rather than their most polished performer. How can you identify such people?

Most people who are prominent in public health advocacy receive virulent and sometimes threatening letters and phone calls from people who oppose their cause. Mostly these are anonymous but when such letters are signed or the callers identify themselves, they can be put to good effect. Rather than discarding these letters or names, keep them on file. Journalists will sometimes ask your advice about potential interviewees who represent an opposite viewpoint to yours. Consider referring journalists to these cranks, taking care to forewarn them that they are likely to find your opposition obnoxious and unintelligent. If

---

Case study: crank letters

The gun lobby in Australia is factionalised into various groups representing different constituencies of shooting interests. All of these groups oppose the main platforms of gun control—for example, bans on semi-automatic weapons, registration of all guns, narrowing of definitions of "need to own" a gun. Some of the groups are adept at identifying themselves with forms of shooting that enjoy considerable social support (such as Olympic pistol shooting). When these groups appear in opposition to gun control advocates, they cloak their arguments in a veneer of respectability that distracts from their affinity with the views of the more aggressive arms of the gun lobby. The opposition to gun control from these other sections of the gun lobby derives from an overt gung-ho "arm the people", jingoistic agenda that alarms many people who might otherwise not feel one way or the other about gun control arguments. The Coalition for Gun Control in Australia generally refers journalists to these more extreme groups for comment.

they are interviewed, the extremism of these people will contrast well with your arguments and demeanour.

Creative epidemiology

Creative epidemiology marries the science of the researcher with the creativity of the media advocate. "Creative epidemiology" is a term coined by Australian public health advocate Mike Daube to describe the process of translating often complicated epidemiological data into terms more easily understood by the media and general public. In practice, it has come to mean the reworking of any complicated or old, time worn data into new, interesting, and arresting forms. It is particularly concerned with placing unfamiliar or complicated data in perspective against data that are more familiar to people. Creative epidemiology can assist in translating the important aspects of research findings to inexpert audiences who may well be mistrustful of data and who are likely to glaze over when statistics are mentioned.

Here are several common ways of expressing epidemiological data "creatively".

- If your annual incidence numbers seem relatively small and unimpressive, consider aggregating them over a longer period. People working in AIDS advocacy, for example, frequently cite the total number of people who have acquired HIV and AIDS since the first cases were diagnosed, whereas reporting of more established diseases is generally expressed in terms of annual incidence of new cases.

  Another aspect of this can be in making the incidence of seemingly unsensational or inconsequential behaviours or exposures appear much more startling. The tobacco industry, for example, may try to insist that urban pollution is of far more consequence to respiratory health than smoking. Many people might find this argument appealing. Using creative epidemiology, you can argue that 20-a-day smokers, inhaling an average of 12 times per cigarette, will pull a carcinogenic smoke cocktail down into their lungs at point blank range some 87 600 times a year ($20 \times 12 \times 365$ days) or 1752 000 times in 20 years. Such a figure places the vague claims about ambient, dissipated, urban pollution in greater perspective.

- Correspondingly, if the numbers you are dealing with are mind bogglingly large, these can sometimes be more dramatically expressed if they are placed in perspective against short time frames. World population control advocates, for example, frequently make statements such as "every day, the population of the world increases by three million" to try and make the hazy implications of world population blowout appear more meaningful. Another example: Sir Patrick Sheehy, head of BAT, the transnational tobacco giant, was described in Britain's *Daily Telegraph* as earning "£19 000 a day" rather than in the annual salary and benefits sum of £6935 000 from which this figure must have been calculated, a figure to which it is much harder to relate.[13]
- When trying to give some sense of meaning to extremely large sums of money—for example, the annual cost of treating a preventable disease—consider translating this sum into how many socially beneficial alternatives this sum could buy, such as how many schools, how many public housing units, how many shelters for the homeless.
- People today are so used to seeing the numbers "million" and "billion" used that they lose their effect, especially when used to describe national or international problems. One strategy to use in overcoming this tendency is to *localise* statistics, calculating, for example, how many people in your area alone are affected by a particular problem, or how much community-wide health problems will cost each citizen. Such calculations often present a new and engaging angle on a seemingly remote story.

Making a story local and personal involves your community in a way that global or national stories rarely can. Even within a good national campaign, much can be done to add local content and perspective—and help create support for local initiatives.

A statistic used in smoking control advocacy campaigns provides an ideal illustration. To ordinary people, 18 000 Australian deaths a year from smoking is less involving than 10 deaths a day in their own city. Local statistics, local role models (such as a local shopkeeper who won't sell cigarettes), or local efforts to change public health policies can seem more

Case study: creative epidemiology

Steve Woodward, formerly Australian director of ASH (Action on Smoking and Health) gathered together others' data on the cigarette brand preferences of Australian children smokers in four different states. Their preferences corresponded perfectly and dramatically with the brands of cigarette that sponsored the major football code played in each of the four states. Woodward had the data made up into a simple graph and distributed it to all politicians and the media (figure 3).

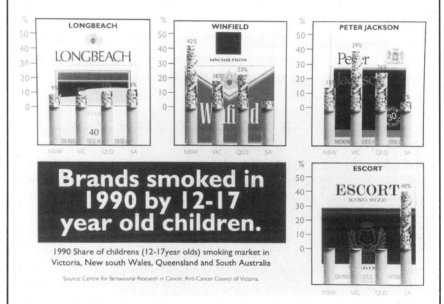

Figure 3: The "graph" that helped to convince the Australian Minister for Sport that tobacco sponsorship had to stop.

The graph and its implications (that the tobacco industry's claim that tobacco sponsorship of football was not a form of advertising, and that even if it was, it did not influence children in any way) became pivotal in the Federal Government's support of a legislative ban on tobacco sponsorship. At the Government's announcement of its intention to introduce the ban, the Minister for Sport, Ros Kelly, said of the graph "This is what influenced me". The graph was reproduced on the front page of Sydney's leading newspaper the following morning.[14]

relevant to your fellow citizens and community leaders than more remote national stories.

- Try to give some *relativity* to numbers by contrasting the new and unfamiliar with the old and familiar. Time-honoured examples here are to compare losses from particular diseases with losses during wars—for example, more people died of gun violence in one week in the United States than occurred to allied forces during the whole period of the Gulf War, the Clinton administration's regular comparison of there being "more gun dealers than gas stations" in the United States. In 1993 on Australia's Cancer Awareness Day, the Australian Prime Minister's wife, Ms Annita Keating, stated that "more [Australian] women die from breast cancer each month than have died from AIDS in the past decade" when calling for more community and government concern about the disease that affects one in every 14 women during their life.

Demonstrations

Well attended demonstrations, pickets, and street marches will nearly always attract media attention by virtue of their sheer size. Small demonstrations can also be newsworthy, however, if they are dramatic or if they involve the participation of people who in some way disturb the usual expectations of who it is that takes part in demonstrations or to whom they are usually directed. Counter-demonstrations can also be newsworthy (*see* Gate-crashing) and can cut into the news time being obtained by the principal demonstration.

There is virtually a genre of demonstration reporting which includes the following elements: a statement of the grievance or purpose causing the demonstration; an estimate of the size of the crowd; shots of placards or banners that have caught the camera operator's eye (usually witty or bordering on the libellous); close ups of any famous or bizarrely dressed people marching or involved in the demonstration; excerpts from speeches made at the demonstration or from interviews with its organisers; comments from the opponents of the demonstration; and comments from passers-by witnessing the demonstration.

Most of these elements can inspire some planning by advocates. Rather than just hoping to leave the positive reporting of a demonstration to luck, thought should be put into the "tone" that you would like to set for the demonstration. If, for example, you sense that your issue is often negatively characterised by the media as one driven by neo-puritans and health zealots, think of ways to project images that belie such assumptions (*risqué* placards, celebrities as spokespeople, etc). During the anti-Vietnam war demonstrations in the 1960s and 1970s in Australia, efforts were made to encourage marchers who were middle aged and elderly to join in: students were urged to coax their parents into marching, and to wear suits. This was an attempt to counter community feelings that anti-war demonstrators were mostly young anarchists who did not represent mainstream Australian society.

An analyst of gay and AIDS activism has written:

There is a fine line between, on the one hand, street theatre, civil disobedience, and the right to demonstrate, and on the other, mob behaviour and brownshirting . . . Many fear that the politics of anger is causing the community to abandon its commitment to the freedom of expression and the right to privacy, the two ideas used most often to support gay rights.[15] [16]

If you believe that your issue is one that will attract very angry people (either on your side or as hecklers and interjectors from your opposition) give strong consideration to whether this aspect of the demonstration has the potential to become the main news angle, replacing the reasons for the demonstration in the way it is reported. If this happens, your demonstration will probably be counterproductive, despite making prime time news (*see* the introduction to Part II).

Here are some considerations to keep in mind when planning demonstrations.

- Inform the media about what your group intends doing in regard to the planned demonstration. Demonstrations can sometimes be short lived if officials require you to leave the scene. It is therefore important that whatever you do occurs when cameras and journalists are present and ready.
- Produce pamphlets, bumper stickers, T-shirts with slogans, banners, and placards. One year, Melbourne MOP UP had a

Case study: demonstrations

In 1985, the Australian Lawn Tennis Association announced that it was ending many years of lucrative sponsorship from Marlboro and joining instead with Ford in staging the Australian Open, part of the prestigious international Grand Slam circuit. For each of the four years previous to the announcement, Melbourne MOP UP (Movement Opposed to the Promotion of Unhealthy Products) had staged demonstrations outside the courts where the tournament was played. On several occasions, high ranking tennis officials spoke to MOP UP demonstrators and said that Marlboro was proving a very embarrassing sponsorship because of all the publicity MOP UP were getting. MOP UP believe it to be no coincidence that Marlboro was dropped following their annual campaign, although of course Philip Morris deny this, explaining their departure in terms of "a purely commercial decision".

Around the same time, two of Australia's most successful motor racing teams voluntarily dropped several million dollars of tobacco sponsorship from Marlboro and Peter Stuyvesant because of anti-smoking feeling in the community. The Mazda team's chief executive said that he didn't want his race team's cars involved with a cigarette company, "Because there is a significant number of people in the community who are hostile to cigarettes and we don't want that hostility to spread to us."[17]

giant inflatable plastic cigarette made up and emblazoned with "Come to Cancer Country" along its length (figure 4). The following year they organised and publicised a mock funeral car procession that would drive to the court area. Some cars were painted black with special wash-off paint, others were daubed with slogans explaining the funeral to onlookers, which included major television stations. Outside the entrance in the car park they assembled a mock graveyard with cardboard box cut-out facsimile headstones saying such things as "Here lies the Unknown Marlboro Cowboy—Saddled with

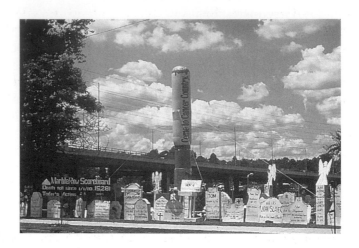

Figure 4: Melbourne MOP UP (Movement Opposed to the Promotion of Unhealthy Products) display outside the tobacco sponsored Australian Open tennis championships.

a Dopey Habit." They even arranged for a light airplane to skywrite "CANCER COUNTRY" in the sky above the courts. As luck would have it, there was no wind and the full wording remained legible for some minutes. Three stickers produced by Melbourne BUGA UP read "JOIN McENROE—BREAK A RACKET. KEEP TOBACCO COMPANIES OUT OF SPORT", "TOBACCO SPONSORSHIP—A PAIN IN THE ARTS", and "MARLBORO TAKES THE WIND OUT OF TENNIS". If your group has little money, the content of pamphlets and slogans on stickers should be general enough to be relevant to different events at which you will be protesting, covering the general theme of your issue—not simply one particular topical issue. If you are in a position to create different material for each event, this is all the better.

- Stage street theatre. London's COUGHIN held a demonstration outside the Royal Festival Hall in August 1985 where the London Festival Ballet were dancing, with the sponsorship of John Player Special cigarettes. Ballet music from a portable cassette was played while Death danced and gave out cigarettes to other COUGHIN dancers who promptly fell about dying, whereupon doctors dressed in white coats, stethoscopes, coloured tights and tutus rushed in with medical help. The ballet fans loved it, took some 1000 leaflets and gave donations.

- Publicise (and maybe even hold) a spoof alternative event to the one about which you are protesting. DOC (Doctors Ought to Care) held the "Emphysema Slims" tennis tournament in Augusta, Georgia, in March 1985 and got the support of a number of celebrities and a lot of press coverage.
- Distribute pamphlets explaining your protest and giving suggestions for action by those who share your concerns.
- Create an alternative prize, which should be displayed to those filing into the arena. Protests inside venues will need to be orderly enough to give the authorities no cause to have you removed. Making any disturbance that distracts players, performers, or delegates and spectators may give your message a short blaze of glory, but result in your ejection, with the incident most likely reported in "rabble-rousing" terms. A better ploy is to engage in passive, less obtrusive forms of protest—for example, if six people can sit in a row together at a tobacco sponsored tennis match, they could wear T-shirts each with the single letters forming "C-A-N-C-E-R" boldly written on them. This will be easily read by all spectators and unavoidably picked up by the television long range shots as part of the background. If you take banners in, give some thought to when you will unfurl them, keeping in mind that you may be asked to take them down.

At the final of the Benson and Hedges cricket cup at Lords in England in 1985, a suitably worded banner was tied to the roof of an adjacent tall building which just happened to contain the apartment of a London activist. It was estimated that some 20 000 people would have been in direct sight of the banner during the full day as well as the television cameras. This was opportunism in full flight!

- Consider entering promotions held by your opposition. Sales promotions disguised as competitions or talent quests are common. Philip Morris held a competition in Australia in 1981 where they sought an Australian Marlboro man with the lure of $25 000 and an advertising contract. The activist group

BUGA UP took a pause from their usual illegal graffiti refacing of outdoor billboard advertisements, and decided to enter someone appropriate in the contest. A man confined to a wheelchair who smoked through his tracheotomy air hole was approached in a Sydney hospital. The man, Frank, agreed to enter the contest as BUGA UP's entrant. Not a group to do things quietly, BUGA UP decided not only to enter the contest formally but also to produce a poster of Frank for placement on the billboards of Sydney. Frank's entry attracted considerable press attention to the point that when the largest selling Sydney morning newspaper reported the eventual contest winner, three out of four newspaper columns were spent describing the BUGA UP entry. The poster was later used on the cover of the *Medical Journal of Australia*.[18]

For some years, the makers of John Player Special cigarettes have sponsored an exhibition for portraiture at London's National Portrait Gallery. In 1984 Bristol AGHAST entered the competition with a portrait by a sympathetic Bristol artist, William Guilding, of a wasted, emaciated man in his early 30s propped up in a hospital bed with an oxygen cylinder. In his hand he held a cigarette. The painting (figure 5) was titled "The early death of Jack Filbert". A slide of the painting was sent for first round judging by the Gallery's staff and short-listed for the second round of judging. At this stage, tobacco chiefs became involved in the selection for exhibition and the painting was shown the door. For reasons known only to them, they decided that this portrait of a smoker dying from lung cancer would not be hung in their tobacco sponsored exhibition.

Like all good campaigners, AGHAST were aware that failures must be turned into successes and so decided to hold an alternative exhibition, titled the Lung Slayer Portrait Award. The footpath outside the National Portrait Gallery seemed as good a place as any to stage the exhibition and the morning of the announcement of the John Player award, when art critics and journalists would be turning up to nibble *hors d'oeuvres*, seemed a suitable time. About eight people staffed the alternative exhibition. A suitable pamphlet was produced, the rejected painting made up into a poster for sale to passers-by and some appropriate banners displayed ("John Slayer

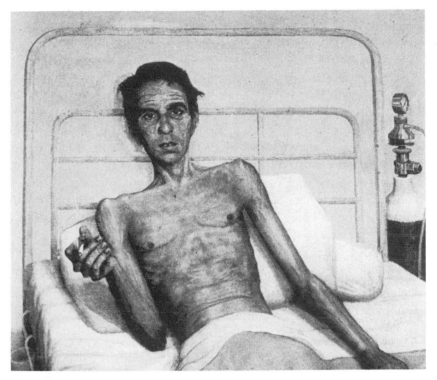

Figure 5: Cover of *The Lung Goodbye*, featuring the painting "The early death of Jack Filbert".

Portraits: In your local cancer ward now!"; "The real sponsors are dying in cancer wards"; "Who put the 'art' in heart disease?"; and "There's no art in drug pushing"). Good press coverage of the alternative award was achieved with the *Guardian* newspaper running a photo of the alternative award but not the tobacco award winner.

Divide and rule

The British colonial empire principle of "divide and rule" has application in advocacy. If your opposition is somehow dis-united on any aspect of the public health issue in question, try to pry open this disunity in any way that will cause them to become sidetracked into squabbling together rather than being more powerfully united in their opposition to your goals.

Beware also of the "divide and rule" principle being used by your opposition to weaken your advocacy efforts. In the context of discussing resource allocations by government to health issues, Wachter warns, "Disease-specific activist groups may find themselves pitted against one another as they advocate their own interests."[20] If you can be sensitive enough to see that such divide and rule equivalents are happening, try to stand back from the foreground conflicts and ask yourself if the issues involved in these are as important as the bigger picture issues that are being neglected because of petty conflicts (*see* the introduction to Part II).

Case study: divide and rule (1)

In 1986, the Philip Morris tobacco company launched a promotional exercise throughout Australia known as the *Peter Jackson Rock Circuit*. It signed up dozens of local rock bands and heavily promoted the concerts and venues where the Rock Circuit would be playing. The exercise was an obvious attempt to associate smoking and the Peter Jackson brand of cigarettes with rock culture.

Phil Thornton, who worked in New South Wales on the "Quit. For Life" campaign, and I, who at the time was working in South Australia, decided to try to use the divide and rule principle to throw the promotion into chaos by fanning the already glowing embers of a divided rock music industry. We contacted several leading rock bands and performers who were not involved in the tobacco circuit and asked them if they were prepared to sign a statement condemning the use of rock musicians to promote tobacco. We had no difficulty in getting support and decided then to publish an advertisement incorporating the signed statement in the national press. Money was paid for the advertisement (figure 6) from our campaign budgets but received publicity far in excess of the advertisement, from the story the issue generated in the wider media. Because the rock bands supporting us included "stars" who were speaking out on a social issue, namely, doing something other than playing music, the media went into a "feeding frenzy" of interviews where the rock stars expressed their views on the issue.

For reasons that were never disclosed, the tobacco promotion simply folded. No tobacco rock promotions have since been held in Australia.

Case study: divide and rule (1) continued

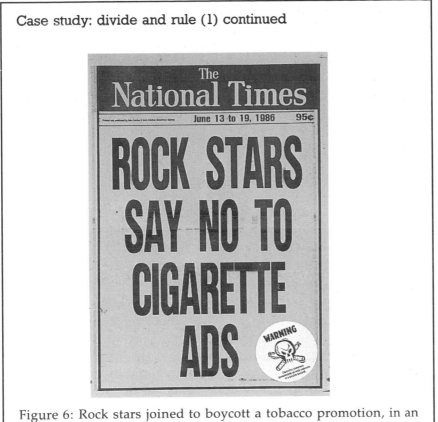

Figure 6: Rock stars joined to boycott a tobacco promotion, in an advertisement in the Australian national press.

Case study: divide and rule (2)

Rugby League, the main professional football code in New South Wales and Queensland, Australia has been sponsored for many years by a Rothmans' tobacco brand, Winfield. The sponsorship has attracted heated criticism from health workers and many members of the public, but the hundreds of players who each week are obliged to assist Rothmans in their promotion are all forbidden under the terms of their contracts to criticise their sponsor. Most of the players do not smoke and, over the years, many have privately expressed their distaste

---

Case study: divide and rule (2) continued

for having to play in a tobacco sponsored competition. In 1991, the NSW Public Health Association sent individual questionnaires to all players in three grades at eight clubs playing in the weekly Winfield Cup competition. They were invited to vote on several questions about the tobacco sponsorship and the desirability of alternative sponsors being found. League officials found out about the poll and threatened players with disciplinary action if they participated in the vote. None the less, 54 out of 400 questionnaires sent out were returned, with 62% of these supporting an alternative sponsor. The League reacted by commissioning its own poll of players, with the predictable result that 67% of players supported Winfield. The League's publicity machine trumpeted this result, but the Public Health Association used its experience of a "censored poll" to divide and rule the issue with the *Sydney Morning Herald*'s lead sporting page headline reading "Health body slams League poll claim".[19]

Doctors

There is a long established historical reluctance among doctors to become involved in any activity that might be construed as publicity. Since Hippocrates, the medical profession has considered that its professionalism has little in common with ventures in the public arena. Hippocrates exhorted physicians to avoid activities that "savour of fuss or show"[21] and in 1905 William Osler advised doctors not to "dally with the Delilah of the press".[22] DeVries reports that, until the late 1970s, some medical students were taught that a doctor's name should appear in the press only at birth, death, and marriage.[23] The *New England Journal of Medicine* explicitly discourages authors appearing in its pages from holding press conferences.[24 25] Consequently, many doctors are highly suspicious of the media and are reluctant to court its attention actively in the ways advocated in this book.

Out of the clinics, surgeries, and operating theatres

On the other hand, doctors can play very powerful roles in media advocacy. Doctors who break out of the sanctum of the doctor–patient relationship and into public health advocacy fascinate the media. Their relationship to patients lends them an authenticity of concern for prevention that is unique and rarely challenged. The subtext of a clinician or "hands-on" doctor speaking out in the media is "here is a person who knows first hand the consequences of the neglect of this public health issue". It is difficult for someone in opposition to a public health initiative to refute or obfuscate the immediate clinical experience of a doctor. If a politician talks about the need to rationalise health services or the waste of taxpayers' money going into duplication of a service, many of the public will acknowledge that this framing of budget cuts to health services makes sense: who could agree with waste and duplication? Statements against such cuts by the political opposition to the government will be dismissed by many as just plain politicking but, if hospital surgeons speak out about the human face of surgical waiting lists, the frame is invariably a more powerful one of "people at the coal-face speaking out about the realities."

Saul Alinsky advised, "Wherever possible go outside of the experience of the enemy."[9] Doctors are extraordinarily capable of doing this whenever they evoke their clinical experience with people afflicted with disease or injuries. If you are a doctor and work in a clinical situation, in debates with your opposition, emphasise how distressing it is to hear your opponent trying to downplay significance of the public health problem. Invite a member of an anti-immunisation group to visit your hospital, for example, and see for themselves children coughing from pertussis. Talk about anti-immunists' insensitivity, their sheltered lives, how cocooned they are from reality.

Doctors are also prized scalps for many of the opponents of public health. There is a saying, "A doubting or smoking doctor is worth $100 000 of free advertising" to the tobacco industry. This is no doubt an apocryphal statement which is passed around in smoking control circles as a piece of lore said to have been uttered by some senior tobacco executive. Its origins are unimportant, but its truth is most certainly salutary. The medical profession has been in the vanguard of smoking control and its collected clinical, pathological, and epidemiological assessment of tobacco's role in ill health continues to be the main reference point in the arguments for smoking control.

In a 1984 edition of the *Medical Journal of Australia*, its then editor wrote an editorial entitled "Smoke gets in your eyes".[26] Several writers pointed out that the piece closely resembled several of the main anthems used by the tobacco industry. It was incredible and terribly disappointing to find such cant in the pages of Australia's leading medical journal. In following editions, some 22 letters condemning the piece and its writer were published. But its value was not lost to the industry. At the time, I predicted that they would engrave its sentiments, fully referenced, into the frontline of their propaganda efforts. As if to oblige, within the year the editorial was being incorporated into the industry's dealings with officialdom, attached as the only appendix in a submission by the Tobacco Institute of Australia to the Broadcasting Review Board of Hong Kong's enquiry into advertising.

Any doctor who overtly or inadvertently supports your opposition should either be quietly but firmly taken aside (if it seems to have been done in ignorance or innocence) or else jumped on from a great height by his or her peers in the medical profession, if the support is plainly deliberate. The public must be left in no doubt that the doctor is unrepresentative of the overwhelming consensus in the profession.

Editorials

All major newspapers print daily editorials. These usually concern major current news stories although editorials about continuing or seasonal issues—for example, the holiday season roll toll, the plight of the homeless during winter months—are also published. Forthcoming important dates, such as World No Tobacco Day, anniversaries of major road disasters, pre-budget periods, can serve as good pretexts to raise particular issues with the press in the hope of attracting an editorial or feature.

Editorials are written by editorial staff employed by a newspaper. These staff may be totally dedicated to editorial writing, or reporters who have been asked to write an editorial based on their recent reporting of an issue. In either case, those writing editorials will be looking for inspiration and material in much the same way that ordinary news reporting occurs. It is common for special interest groups to approach newspapers with requests that editorials be written.

Before you approach newspaper editorial representatives, make sure you know what their paper has written on your subject in the past. If you are going to ask a newspaper to take a particular stand on an issue, you should know what the paper has already said about it. It will also help you tailor your case to the special interests of your target audience. Some organisations keep files on what their local papers have written on issues of importance to them. Such a filing system can be very useful in preparing for discussions with representatives of the papers.

Editorial memoranda

An editorial memorandum is a detailed explanation of a particular position on a particular issue that should be sent to the editor. The tone of an editorial memorandum (memo) should be thoughtful and reasoned. Although an editorial memo takes an unapologetically partisan approach to a topic, it should not be as strident as a piece of political propaganda, such as a leaflet or partisan speech.

An editorial memo should be sent out with a cover letter that clearly states the position the memo advocates. The memo itself can be several pages long and should clearly spell out all of the major arguments supporting the stated position. Significant supporting evidence, such as articles or studies, can be attached as appendices. The memo should also anticipate major counter-arguments to your position and provide an adequate response.

Keep in mind that a good editorial memo should serve as a primary resource for the journalist who wants to write an editorial endorsing your position. Therefore, editorial memos are best produced by a peak policy body, national organisation or other reputable group of people. Newspaper editors who receive a memo will want to know without doubt that the information contained within the memo is current and accurate. An editorial memo should never be thought of as a replacement for personal contact. Even if your editorial memo contains every good argument that exists in favour of your position, a personal meeting with an editorial representative will greatly enhance your chances for success.

Elitism

Many public health workers are middle class, well educated people whose own high brow media habits place them in stark contrast with those of most of the population. It is not uncommon to hear people in public health being disdainful of the quality of populist media and being averse to watching, listening, and reading it. Such attitudes can sometimes translate into an ill advised neglect of the importance of populist media as vehicles for media advocacy discourses.

Mark Ragg, a freelance medical writer for Australian newspapers, makes the point, somewhat exaggerated but worth reflection:

Politicians do not care what the so-called "quality press" says about them, because the "quality press" is constitutionally anti-politician and anti-government. It is the popular media, which are usually less critical, which have far more influence in swaying a politician's thinking. The thinking, an odd mixture of elitism and realism, is that any thoughtful person is going to dislike most government decisions, so we may as well try to influence the less thoughtful ones who buy the tabloid newspaper and who watch tabloid television.[27]

Whatever the accuracy of this reflection, advocates should think about whether their own media preferences are biasing their objective assessment of how best to target particular media. If populist media are considered important to your campaign, you may need to swallow your pride and get into the habit of regularly reading newspapers written for the lowest common denominator, or listening to tedious and irritating radio programmes, to enable you to judge how to pitch an upcoming interview. If you are going to be interviewed for a particular radio or television programme, it is imperative that you familiarise yourself with it before you do the interview. Assess the style of the interviewer; the length of the interviews; the length of the "bites" or "grabs" if it is an edited programme; whether it is a "serious" or light programme and so on (*see* Interview strategies).

Facsimile machines

A facsimile (fax) machine can immeasurably improve the ability of advocacy groups to access the media. Access to a fax during both business and after hours is important—no—read *essential*. A home fax allows rapid responses to be made to news that breaks overnight, during weekends, and holiday periods. Morning radio and television news editors will often be searching for commentary and follow up stories on news that has broken late on the previous day or overnight when many office-hours spokespeople cannot be reached. A press release commentary faxed to radio and television stations late at night will be waiting for the crews who assemble the morning news programmes early that day. They will often be grateful to have someone offering to comment on a story, rather than having to wake up a potential commentator who may not be aware of the news incident in question, who may be unavailable or unprepared. Be sure to have either a supply of your group's stationery at home, or software that allows you to print your letterhead using a home computer.

Fact sheets

Succinct, comprehensive, and journalist friendly fact sheets are an invaluable part of advocacy work. Most journalists have educational backgrounds in the humanities, not the sciences, and consequently can be awed or intimidated by health and medical issues.[28] Succinct summaries and demystified background material on public health issues will often be gratefully snapped up by journalists who feel a little at sea about your issue. Fact sheets should be written with particular readers in mind—for example, students, politicians, journalists, volunteers, and fund-raisers, or the general public. The content, style, and comprehensiveness of the sheets will vary according to what you understand to be the typical information needs and existing awareness of your target audience.

It is often a good idea to set out fact sheets in a question and answer format, anticipating the issues with which your target group may be preoccupied. The questions you select can be a mixture of the questions that you know are the most commonly asked by (say) journalists; those that address the main arguments put forward by your opposition (remember that journalists seeking "balance" will often want to see where you stand in relation to your opposition's main arguments); and those questions that frame your position best, allowing you to position particular perspectives that may not have received wide coverage.

It is often a good idea to include references to the facts and claims made in such material. Referencing gives such material more of an appearance of authority and credibility.

Case study: fact sheets

In October, 1992, a representative of the powerful United States National Rifle Association was due to visit Australia at the invitation of the local pro-gun lobby. On learning of this, Rebecca Peters of the Coalition for Gun Control put together a comprehensive fact sheet which addressed all the arguments that the gun lobby use as well as all the platforms of a comprehensive gun control policy. The fact sheet, together with lists of expert commentators on most aspects of gun control (comparative international law, the police, domestic violence, the banking industry, psychiatry, community physicians, and surgeons), were sent to all media outlets. The Coalition members were inundated with calls from a grateful media who clearly found the material user friendly and accessible, with various reports making it evident that journalists had directly lifted questions and slices of text from the material provided.

Fillers

Radio stations frequently require material to fill short gaps in their programming: items that radio announcers can turn to when they have 15 seconds or so between the end of a piece of music and a scheduled news bulletin, for example. You can exploit this need by supplying radio announcers or station management with short items that take only a few seconds to read. These can be set out in lists under your topic (for example, "Amazing but true facts about [your issue]"; "20 advances in injury prevention in the last decade") or you can fax individual fillers to the radio station when they are topical around, say, a world or national [disease] day.

Gatecrashing

Your opposition will almost certainly hold functions, ceremonies, press conferences, public meetings, prize givings, and sponsored events where your group's presence will be most unwelcome. These events will often attract huge media coverage and be attended by people you seek to influence or wish to draw out on an issue. Your presence at the event may cause a valuable split in the media coverage given to it. Instead of one-sided reports focusing on your opposition's claims or activities at their meeting, media stories on the event will cover your presence and arguments too, often halving your opposition's media coverage. The party the organisers meant to hold may not turn out to be the party that they get. In recent years, every annual international AIDS conference has featured demonstrations at the opening session by ACT UP, causing the international media to focus as much attention on the demonstration and its rationale as on the opening session.

Case study: gatecrashing

BUGA UP, the Australian anti-tobacco graffiti group, gatecrashed an international conference of advertising agencies held at the Sydney Opera House in 1986. The group constructed a makeshift "confessional" booth out of a simple frame, curtains, and two chairs (figure 7). They had one of their members dress up in ecclesiastical costume. He approached delegates as they made their way into the conference. A sign above the booth urged advertisers who worked on tobacco accounts and who wrote sexist advertising copy to come into the booth and confess their "sins". The booth was immensely popular with many of the delegates who took it in good humour, and immensely annoying and embarrassing to others. The booth split the Sydney media's coverage of the conference, effectively seizing some of the agenda in a way never intended by the conference organisers.

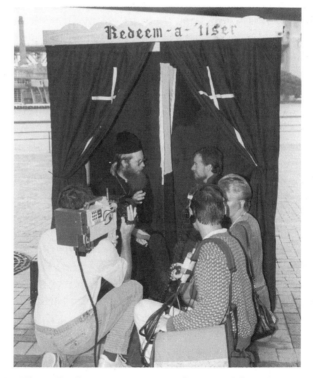

Figure 7: The "Redeem-a-'tiser confessional booth" outside the 1986 advertising conference in Sydney.

Infiltration

If your group poses a serious threat to your opposition, it is certain that they will attempt to gain as much intelligence about you as possible (*see* Know your opposition). They will endeavour to obtain any newsletters or publications you produce (*see* Mailing lists), attend all public meetings you call and may try to tap your phones and even infiltrate your organisation using "spies" disguised as interested citizens.

Community groups that operate with volunteers and accordingly do not run reference checks or other authenticating procedures on their staff may be vulnerable to such infiltration. Similarly, if you are organising meetings or conferences where you hope for, and expect, open discussion of strategy and planning among like minded colleagues, attendance at such events will be very tempting to your opposition. Recent World Conferences on Tobacco and Health held in Perth, Australia, and Buenos Aires have endeavoured to exclude any representatives from the tobacco or allied industries. Perth was largely successful in this policy, whereas Buenos Aires failed dismally: tobacco industry operatives sat in on all sessions that promised even a whiff of revelation about strategy. The resulting atmosphere was understandably charged, suspicious, and stilted.

If you wish to exclude your opposition from public meetings or conferences, you should indicate this on any announcements or registration brochures, and require people to indicate their affiliation when they register. Suspicious looking registrants can then be scrutinised in advance. Door registrations can leave you more vulnerable, especially in the busy, chaotic periods when registration staff do not have the time to check details. If you suspect that someone in a seminar or meeting is an operative, you can ask all the registrants to introduce themselves and say where they are from. If someone sounds doubtful, your next step may be to politely confront the person with your suspicions, explaining the sensitive nature of the meeting, and that "no one else here seems to know you, so you'll understand that we are concerned."

There are ways that you can "infiltrate" your opposition too. One way is to send "freelance journalists" to interview your opposition. Journalists regularly call or visit businesses and

181

Case study: infiltration

In the early 1980s, BUGA UP, the Australian anti-tobacco billboard graffiti group, was infiltrated by a man, John, who posed as someone who had long admired their work and wanted to assist. He assisted in driving BUGA UP members around to billboards and was very keen to do whatever he could. After a television programme had run a major item on the anti-smoking movement in Australia, four activists' houses were spray painted the next day. A BUGA UP meeting was called to discuss tactics in dealing with the issue. John attended and offered to drive around to each house which had been defaced, and to photograph the damage. As the details of this were being discussed and John was being given all the addresses of the houses, another BUGA UP member joined the meeting saying that her neighbour had taken the details of a car driving slowly up her street and photographing the sprayed fence. The licence plate had been noted and the car turned out to be John's. He was confronted, and admitted he was an infiltrator, although refused to say who he was working for.

Case study: infiltration

David Sweanor, a lawyer and Canadian tobacco control advocate, once visited the Tobacco Institute in Australia unannounced. He said he was a lawyer with an interest in tobacco regulation (true!) and was visiting Sydney and wanted to take the opportunity to see how the issues differed in Australia from Canada (again true!). He was able to interview an unsuspecting executive who opened up in revealing detail about how the industry saw the future, which initiatives it feared the most and who it saw as its main enemies. That afternoon, the information was passed to local tobacco control advocates who couldn't believe their luck.

community organisations involved in topical issues, in an attempt to gather information or interviews for potential reports. In my academic work, I have set assignments for students to analyse public health issues from the perspective of both public health advocates and their opposition. This has sometimes inspired students to try to interview (for example) tobacco industry executives and sometimes they have succeeded, returning assignments that include most interesting tape-recorded material full of candid information.

Interview strategies*

Many public health workers would have spent many hundreds of hours during their careers preparing presentations such as lectures and speeches for students, conferences, and community meetings. The biggest of such occasions might be a national or international conference, where perhaps several thousand people might be listening to a plenary presentation in a huge auditorium. The far more common presentation will be to a room full of students, colleagues, or consumers. Such occasions set up expectations that speakers will be suitably prepared, that they will have objectives, a planned beginning, middle, and end to their speech or lecture, that they will have suitable slides or visual aids, that they will have rehearsed their presentation with colleagues, and so on. Awareness of these expectations often drives speakers and lecturers into lengthy preparation.

The contrast of such nth degree preparation with the typical preparation made for a news interview is invariably stark. The best example from my own experience occurred when I was working in New Delhi, India, in 1985. I had been asked to give a talk on tobacco control strategies to workers from the Voluntary Health Association of India. I delivered a well prepared talk in a stifling lecture theatre in a university to perhaps 30 people. Immediately afterwards, I was approached by a young man with a tape recorder who politely asked if I had a few moments to give

* Entire books and training programmes have been devoted to this area. One of the best books I have read in this area is by Sarah Dickinson (*How to take on the media*, London: Weidenfeld & Nicholson, 1990).

a short interview for his radio station. I was late for another appointment, but obliged. At the end of our impromptu, casual chat I asked him what radio station he worked for. He worked for the central government broadcasting service and blithely informed me that the interview would be played the next day after the main news bulletins to an estimated listening audience of 200 million!

Such an example highlights the often casual and unprepared way that public health advocates approach opportunities to speak to unparalleled numbers of people, numbered among whom are often many hundreds of significant policymakers and politicians. This section outlines some of the more important strategies that should be considered when being interviewed or when debating in the mass media.

There is a whole industry dedicated to training people (usually from industry and government and usually at great expense) to "perform" better on the media. There is a smaller industry involved in publishing information of the sort that follows. If you expect to be interviewed a great deal by the media, consider investing in one of these courses. Ask other advocates if they can recommend a suitable agency or course.

There are three sorts of interviews that all media advocates will encounter.

- The spur of the moment, unannounced phone call from a print or radio journalist who wants comment immediately. In the case of radio, this may mean that they will ask if they can roll the tape and, within minutes, what you say may be broadcast into millions of homes and cars.
- A prerecorded radio or television interview. These will typically be edited or reduced in length to fit into the news format in which they will be broadcast.
- A live to air radio or television interview, where everything you say, warts and all, will be broadcast.

There are many tips that are worth noting for all three types of interview, while each of them also has its own particular nuances which require forethought. It is essential that you prepare for all of these occasions.

When a journalist phones and you're unprepared

If a print or radio journalist telephones and asks for a comment, it can often happen that you are caught unprepared: that you cannot immediately think of anything worthwhile to say or you do not have the relevant facts at your fingertips. In these situations, buy some time to think it over. Make an excuse—for example, you are with someone, or you need to look up a reference, and promise that you will call back within 10 minutes. This will allow you time to consider your response, to frame it correctly and to work it into a sound bite or compelling quote (see below). Only in rare, "red hot news" situations will a journalist see such a request as unreasonable.

The Advocacy Institute offers the following advice about media performances.

- Don't debate or even think about winning the wrong fight. Your opposition can be maddeningly provocative. Their claims and accusations may sting so sharply that an advocate is drawn into elaborate denials or quibbling over side issues. Ignore the provocations and return to your strong themes and moral high ground.
- Wordiness/mouthfuls. You are trying to persuade a general audience, not impress an audience of your scholarly peers. Do not ramble. Stay with one or two clear points at a time. Do not filibuster; come up for air. Let your opponent get a few words in edgeways.
- Wasting opportunities/getting drawn off track. There's a danger in getting too comfortable with a charming and gracious interviewer and getting drawn off into an interesting side issue that does not advance your policy goals. You may think you've got all the time in the world, but even an hour long talk show can pass by so quickly that you lose the opportunity to hammer home your main points.
- Being unprepared. This needs no explanation.
- Being overprepared. If your words and mannerisms sound memorised or rehearsed, they lose much of their effectiveness. Your arguments and main points should be thoroughly worked out ahead and comfortable, but not in rigid formulas committed to memory.
- Relying on one's status or credentials. If you think that a

sceptical host or a paid industry spokesperson will treat you respectfully because you have an impressive curriculum vitae or are a high ranking executive of a prestigious organisation, think again. Television and radio programming does not favour status or credentials alone. On the other hand, if you are prepared to speak knowledgeably and with authority, then your credentials will help contrast and expose the "hired gun" status of your adversary.

• Mistaking cuteness and sarcasm for wit and humour. Wit and humour are wonderful weapons to disarm a sceptical host or hostile adversary, but not every would-be humorist is good at it. Do not reach for humour or sardonic slogans or labels unless unbiased friends or colleagues confirm that you're good at it. Otherwise, be serious and straight. It's safer.

The Advocacy Institute suggests the following preparation before the programme.

• Find out all you can about the ground rules. What's the format? Who will moderate? Who else will appear on the programme? If this is a regular talk show or interview, try to watch it ahead of time or find colleagues who watch it regularly who can give you a feeling for its norms. Is the host interested in civil discourse or in provoking conflict and confrontation? What expectations do viewers have? Is it the equivalent of the Roman Colosseum or is it a serious minded, background briefing programme where slogans and adversarial talk will sound out of place?

If you can't get the answers to these questions, or if you are uncomfortable with the answers you do get, reconsider whether appearing will serve your goals. If the deck is stacked—the host biased, the questions likely to be ill framed, the "culture" of the show too high powered or trivial for your comfort—pass it up. Not all exposure is good exposure.

• Narrowcast. Ask yourself, who is going to hear or see me? What do you want them to take away from the programme? How do you want to change their attitudes? What do you want them to do?

• You should plan in advance the main points you want to get across sometime during the interview. Ask how long the segment or show is going to run. If you only have three minutes (not unusual on television interviews), concentrate on only one or two key points. If you have longer, you may want

---

Case study: interview strategies

In 1992, Robert Corbin, head of the US National Rifle Association, visited Australia as guest of the gun lobby. At four hours' notice, I was invited to debate with Corbin on Australia's leading current affairs news programme, *A Current Affair*. I was relatively new to the gun control debate and had never seen Corbin on television before. My colleagues and I decided that to refuse the debate would have been handing Corbin a gift to pursue a benign agenda about guns in Australia—to put the best face possible on the issue. We met for an hour before the prerecording time to work out an interview strategy. We had been compiling a list of common frames that the gun lobby uses (guns are important in self defence in the troubled times we live in; people who oppose guns are wimps—the sort who meekly hand over their money to criminals or submit to assault rather than fight back; and that only criminals use guns irresponsibly). Our choice was either to *react* to these sort of framings or to take the offensive and portray Corbin as a representative of an "evil empire" of gun toting rednecks. *A Current Affair* thrives on conflict and good versus evil stories. Accordingly, we saw little point in trying to debate the finer points of gun control policy, but to see the debate as an obvious contest where there would be a winner and loser.

We elected to run with two main themes: firstly, that Corbin was from the United States, well known as the world's capital for gun massacres and drive-by shootings and that his visit to Australia was like inviting an arsonist to give advice on fire control. This framing allowed me to roll off statistics on Australia's comparatively small gun violence problem and to contrast this with the American situation.

Secondly, I decided to portray Corbin as a wolf in sheep's clothing: to contrast his polished and moderate demeanour with the lobbying objectives his organisation pursued in the United States (legalisation of military assault rifles for citizen use and for armour piercing "cop killer" bullets). Fundamentally, my main message was: "Yankee go home—we don't want your advice here when you come from the country with an atrocious record of gun violence."

to add some key supporting arguments or data, but you probably can't effectively convey more than two main themes.

- Outline your points on a single piece of paper. Have it handy so you can glance at it during a break (or whenever necessary if on radio). After the break emphasise the points you have not yet made.

Broadcast appearances are not formal debates scored on the basis of arguing points won or lost. Instead, you must pursue two simultaneous objectives.

- To be persuasive on the issues that you have decided to pursue.
- To make certain that your audience feels that you are a person they like and trust.

Identify the ethical bottom line of your argument

Many viewers, listeners, or readers will be only marginally aware of, or interested in, your issue. Part of the way, however, in which they assess whether they are on your "side" in an advocacy debate will be determined by the extent to which they are able to identify with your "ethical bottom line". Public health issues generally have fairly obvious moral and ethical dimensions to them: protection of the innocent; the rights to information, safety, redress, and justice; community health versus company profits and so on. It is important that you are aware of this dimension to your issue and that you use language which either explicitly or implicitly underscores your message with its ethical conclusions.

Authenticity

Audiences watching or listening to media interviews will be particularly attuned to the extent to which you appear "real" or authentic when being interviewed. Public health advocates often argue for policy changes that are easily characterised by their opponents as work of the "dead hand" of regulatory bureaucracy or government. A common tactic of those who are often being opposed in public health debates is to try to paint you and your group in some calculatingly pejorative way (meddlers, busy-bodies, warriors against pleasure, zealots, even people who would like to adjust the temperature of your shower if they had the chance).[29] Often these frames will succeed in capturing an audience's understanding of who they think you are and what you stand for. It is thus important for you to find ways of making what you are saying sound "authentic"—that you are personally committed to what you are saying—and not that you are merely mouthing the words of a dutiful employee or spokesperson for a committee's policy. Speaking in the first person and being anecdotal are two ways of doing this. Another is to "personalise" your arguments.

Personalising

Saul Alinsky advised that advocates should: "Pick the target, freeze it, personalise it, and polarise it."[9] Your opposition can be conceived of in terms of its policies, its actions, and its consequences for your issue. But such analyses often fail to take account of another way that the community perceives issues: as metaphorical battles between individuals representing particular values. When you appear on television speaking about your public health issue, only a fraction of the viewing audience will attend to what you are saying with anything remotely like the detail you might hope (see Chapter 2). Nearly everyone watching though, will form some opinion about you and your opposition's qualities as human beings. You will evoke a response from the range of very ordinary, everyday human reactions that we all have towards others.

As we noted in Chapters 2 and 3, personalisation is common in health news stories. Many public health issues readily lend themselves to intensely personal framings in ways with which audiences can readily identify: a child burnt and disfigured by unsafe, inflammable nightwear catching fire could so easily be your own; a shopper shot by a gunman going berserk in a state with lax gun laws could so easily be you or your family; it could be your 12 year old child to whom that shop is so willing to sell cigarettes. Try to frame your concerns in these personally relevant sorts of ways rather than as statistical or clinical abstractions.

Case study: interview strategies: personalising

STAT (Stop Teenage Addiction to Tobacco) ran this advertisement (figure 8) in the *Washington Post* on 7 October 1993. It sought to break through the anonymity of corporate respectability by publishing the photographs of five directors of tobacco companies and publishers who run tobacco advertising. It pointed out that not one of them smoked.

Tobacco is an addictive drug — as addictive as heroin.*
Tobacco addiction is America's leading cause of preventable death.*

Meet five of America's richest drug pushers.

Si Newhouse

He could voluntarily refuse to push tobacco in his magazines, as many major magazines do. But he hasn't. His magazines probably do more to make smoking seem attractive and sophisticated — what every young person wants to be — than any others. *Fortune* puts his net worth at $5 billion.

Rupert Murdoch

Tobacco advertising is banned on TV, so tobacco companies go after kids in Murdoch's *TV Guide*. He could say no. He's worth $3 billion.

Larry Tisch

As the man who controls Lorillard Tobacco, he could ask Congress to halt all tobacco advertising and promotion. The tobacco companies would save $4 billion a year. That's $4 billion more annual profit for their shareholders — in the short run. In the long run, fewer kids would be enticed to replace smokers who die or quit. But is that bad? *Fortune* says Tisch is a billionaire.

Henry Kravis

Since his company, RJR, began using a cartoon character to push Camels, Camel's share of the teen and pre-teen market has jumped from 1% to 32%. He could become a health hero by joining with Tisch in asking Congress to ban all tobacco promotion — and boost the industry bottom line by $4 billion. Judging from the *Forbes* 400 list, he can afford this risk. He's worth half a billion.

Michael Miles

Miles runs Philip Morris. Who'd have more reason to want a total ad ban than the shareholders of Philip Morris? Marlboro smokers wouldn't quit buying Marlboros just because the advertising stopped; yet Philip Morris could quit spending all those billions trying to defend its market share. Miles — who himself quit smoking long ago — made $5 million last year.

> What do all five of these men have in common?
> Like most drug pushers, they're smart enough not to use the product they sell. Not one of them smokes cigarettes.

Si, Rupert, Larry, Henry, Mike: If you'll agree it's crazy for a society to *promote* its leading cause of preventable death, and stop doing it, we'll take out an ad **twice as big** honoring you and saying thanks. There's no greater contribution you could make to America's health.

*U.S. Surgeon General

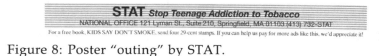

STAT *Stop Teenage Addiction to Tobacco*
NATIONAL OFFICE 121 Lyman St, Suite 210, Springfield, MA 01103 (413) 732-STAT
For a free book, KIDS SAY DON'T SMOKE, send four 29-cent stamps. If you can help us pay for more ads like this, we'd appreciate it!

Figure 8: Poster "outing" by STAT.

As well as addressing your opposition as (say) industry officials or politicians, in public debate address them in their roles as parents, citizens, and human beings. This can dramatically reframe the platform from which they speak and create awkward and telling connotations. Remember always that audiences often attend far more to the subtexts of news items and debates than to the overt content.

During the programme

- Don't be passive or over polite. Interrupt if your opponent is dominating the discussion, but try to do so in a manner that suggests an easy, conversational disagreement rather than hectoring, lecturing, or a panicked feeling overcoming you.
- If your opponent is being obviously rude and domineering, it is likely that many viewers or listeners will be preoccupied with this rather than with what he or she is saying. Quickly and calmly point this rudeness out. This will often trip up your opponent momentarily, allowing you to gain a debating advantage.
- Dress appropriately for the programme on which you are appearing.
- Be simple, clear, and direct. Purge your language of professional jargon and such special shorthand language as the organisational anagrams that those working on an issue are likely to adopt—almost without realising that the rest of the world does not know what they are talking about.
- If you've been distracted and have not heard a question, or if you simply need more time to think, don't be afraid to ask the questioner to repeat the question. But try not to let your mind wander! Time is precious in such settings.
- Use vivid language, colourful illustrations, and be enthusiastic. But above all, be yourself.
- Be sure what you assert as fact is indeed fact. It is better to say nothing than to stretch the truth and be caught out. Don't be afraid to say you do not know the answer to a specific question, or that you are not certain of a specific fact.
- Avoid "trading" scientific studies. This can go on indefinitely and the audience is never sure who has access to the most reliable and important studies.

191

Practise being interviewed

There are commercial "interview schools" in many countries which specialise in training people to be interviewed to their best advantage. These schools are often run by ex-journalists and tend to service political and corporate clients who usually have lots of money to pay for such training. Public health groups are seldom numbered among their clients.

Local community (non-commercial) radio stations typically have very small audiences, yet their radio journalists are often very eager to cover public health stories. It is tempting to think that the time it can take to provide interviews for such stations is hardly worth the effort. In terms of the small audience this may be true; however, the stations can provide you with invaluable practice at being interviewed: if you give a poor performance, few will have heard and you will be the wiser for the next interview opportunity.

Rehearse with colleagues before you are to be interviewed. Get them to role play as host and opponent. Do not memorise answers or points—they will sound memorised. There is a paradox: we all seek the perfect bite (see below). But if it sounds more like a canned slogan than a spontaneous utterance, it loses its effect, especially if it is stale, or an overused cliché.

Media bites or grabs

Knowing your issue in the detail that you do, it may well loom before you as complicated, complex, and inextricably convoluted. Many public health issues *do* have extremely complex aspects to them. If you cannot move past such a perspective on the problems of your area, however, your success as an advocate will be very limited. A critical ability that every public health advocate must possess is to be able to evaluate the essence of the problem that they are dealing with and to translate this essence into small, memorable elements that can be consumed by the media and their audiences. Such elements are known as media bites or grabs. They are short, pithy quotes that serve as a central, characterising feature of a broadcast (sound bites) or print news story. Essentially, they are attention-getting statements that have struck the news editor who cuts your interview down to useable length as being pivotal, emblematic, or simply arresting in some way.

With rare exceptions, radio and television news bulletins are always prerecorded: only very occasionally, such as when the bulletin cuts to a reporter on the spot at a major news event, will live interviews be broadcast. This means that interviews you give for news bulletins will be edited to fit the format of the news bulletin. Table VII shows the length of all news stories run on a randomly selected prime time evening news bulletin on an Australian television channel in February 1993. Apart from advertising and "coming up" announcements, there were 19 stories in a 30 minute bulletin. These stories ran for an average of 66.8 seconds (range 2 minutes 19 seconds to a mere 13 seconds). "Talking heads" of "news actors" were shown 21 times in these stories, with the average talking time being 7.8 seconds.

The obvious lesson here for any interview you give is that you have very little time—a few seconds and perhaps one or two sentences at most—to make the most important points that you hope will be broadcast. The situation with current affairs interview programmes or longer documentaries is considerably different, particularly if the interview is live.

At best, the media bite can serve to encapsulate both information and effective symbols for an audience that is increasingly used to quick bursts of information. A bite can compress your position in a quick, succinct, or witty manner—capturing the attention of the media and the eventual consumer of the message. Like them or not, media bites are a central tool of media advocacy—ignore the "art" of producing good ones at your own loss.

It is not easy to define the qualities that make a successful media bite but here are some suggestions from the Advocacy Institute:

- Use concrete images that evoke a lively response, ones that are fresh, alive, and surprising.
- Avoid sloganeering, shrillness, and moralising.
- Stay brief, and divide longer ideas into short sentences.
- Humour is permissible, but avoid cuteness or frivolity that can downplay the seriousness of the problem. In competing for limited space or time, it is often the pithy or witty quote that gets included in the story. A well conceived quip can deflate

Table VII: Channel 7 news (Sydney) 26 February 1993

Story	Time (min.s)	News actors	Time (s)
73 y old man rapes 9 y old girl	2.06	Psychologist	8
		Friend	8
		Doctor	3
		Politician	9
		Politician	7
Murder charge	1.34	None	N/A
Election: industrial relations	2.03	Opposition leader	2
		Prime Minister	13
		Prime Minister	11
		Prime Minister	6
		Opposition leader	8
Car window tinting to be banned	1.30	Worker	5
		Politician	11
		Industry representative	9
Australian cricket captain sets world record	2.19	Cricketer	12
		Wife	7
		Mother	3
		Wife	3
		Cricketer	15
Floods in Kimberly region	0.29	None	N/A
QE2 ocean liner arrives	1.34	Ship Captain	8
		Passenger	3
		Passenger	5
Somalian aid effort	0.36	None	N/A
Pope meets boxer	0.20	None	N/A
Goods and Service Tax background	1.55	None	N/A
SPORT: More on cricketer's record	1.43	None	N/A
Interstate cricket	0.13	None	N/A
Golf	1.13	None	N/A
Long jump	0.50	None	N/A
World youth soccer cup	0.24	None	N/A
Finance	0.16	None	N/A
Weather	0.45	None	N/A
What's on this weekend	1.00	None	N/A
TV crew visits school	0.20	None	N/A
Mean time	1.7		7.8
Range	2.19–0.13		

N/A = not applicable.

even your opposition's most carefully crafted attempt at legitimacy. Biting humour can also be effective in conveying an appropriate sense of outrage.

- Standard literary devices such as alliteration, rhyming, analogy, parallelism, puns and the like can make a bite resonate with the journalist and the audience.
- Ironic rephrasing of your opposition's statements or popular maxims can contribute to a printable bite. For example, the advertising industry constantly sings the praises of its "self-regulatory" system of advertising standards. By regularly referring to self-regulation as "*shelf*-regulation", public health advocates in Australia have been able economically to underline one of their major criticisms of the system: that complaints from the public are frequently shelved and ignored.
- Remember, the goal is not to earn yourself applause or laughs, but to advance your media advocacy goals.

Some memorable sound bites

- "They've discovered a vaccine against lung cancer and have flushed it down the toilet." (Stan Glantz commenting on the Californian Governor's decision to cut the State's anti-smoking media campaign.)
- "Our cricket authorities have the ethics of a cash register." (Michael Carr-Gregg, after a member of the Australian cricket team was censured and fined by national cricket authorities for having made an anti-smoking advertisement directed at children (Australian cricket is sponsored by the *Benson and Hedges* cigarette brand).)
- "Asking kids to 'say no to drugs' is about as realistic as telling a person with depression to 'have a nice day'." (Criticism made of the naivety of Nancy Reagan's anti-drugs slogan.)

Jargon and ghetto language

Many communications from public health activists suffer from being constipated by a language that seems natural to them, but which is confusing and alienating to many members of the public. Often this language is jargon—words and expressions that are the technical or specialised language of branches of medicine and public health. Sometimes it is also "ghetto language"—a branch of jargon that is developed by groups or causes which typically have a highly refined and politicised sense of their oppression. Ghetto language is often highly politically correct and wanders about in notions of history and knowledge which are taken for granted but which can lose many potential listeners or readers.

Perhaps the main source of lapses into jargon is the classic mistake of confusing your public health objectives with your media objectives (*see* introduction to Part II). As someone working within a complicated area of public health, for example, you may be constantly aware that greater attention to coordination of policies and programmes is required to effect improvements in your public health goal. "Coordination" may well be one of your public health objectives, but as a peg for media interest it is a kiss of death. The term "coordination" is hopelessly vague to members of the public who will generally not have the insights into the problem that you have. They will be attending to what you say, seeking to understand the problem you are expressing in terms of tangible issues with which they can relate. In this example, improved coordination will mean something practical and concrete. It is this that you should talk about in media interviews, not the bureaucratic means of achieving it.

A few examples of public health jargon foisted too often on the public include:

- Utilisation (use)
- Proactive (active)
- Intersectoral (people from different parts of government and the community)
- Liaising (meeting)
- Cohort (group)
- Substance use (drug use)
- Policy.

Of this last, to many people, a "policy" is something they receive each year from their insurance company. They are not used to thinking of public health issues as reflecting "policies". Having a policy enacted may be your preoccupation, but the news listening or newspaper reading public will find discussion of the issue much more accessible if you address the reason for, or the intended effects of, the policy, rather than what sounds like some dull bureaucratic process.

Know your opposition

The more that you know about your opposition, the less likely it will be that you will be disadvantaged being caught unprepared to deal with any tactic or strategy that they use. Knowing the way that your opposition thinks, its preoccupations, strengths, weaknesses, and Achilles heels, and relevant information about its principal members will also allow you to be more strategic in your approach to undermining its public and political support.

You should subscribe or somehow get on the mailing list for all magazines, journals, newsletters, and bulletins published by your opposition (*see* Mailing lists). Campaigners against fluoridation and immunisation, and quack cancer cure groups, for example, regularly spell out their beliefs through "natural health" publications available through newsagents, health food shops, and alternative medicine outlets. The gun lobby has its own publications, usually available through newsagents, with advertisements in these for newsletters available on subscription. The anti-motor cycle helmet lobby often proselytises through biker magazines. The tobacco industry is served by several international trade journals which regularly feature interviews, reports, and information that is indispensable to anyone wanting an inside view of the industry's preoccupations.

Open and maintain active files on your opposition. These might include details of their personnel and leadership, their annual reports, their leading shareholders, other products in their portfolio, outstanding gaffes they may have made, and so on. These files will provide a rich source of information that may trigger useful opportunities when you debate with them or are preparing submissions, etc.

Case study: learning from other campaigners

In 1993 in Australia, governments and health advocates began taking a fresh look at the problem of shopkeepers who sell cigarettes to children. Colleagues in the United States were well advanced of Australia in addressing this problem with research, advocacy, and legal solutions. Dave Altman of Stanford University was contacted and brought to Australia for a national seminar where the lessons learned in America were truncated into a series of recommendations that almost certainly saved local Australian health workers months, if not years, of learning from mistakes already made and corrected in the United States. Sensing that a serious momentum was building against this lucrative source of sales, the Australian tobacco industry began systematically lobbying Government to have them endorse an industry sponsored retailer programme known as "It's the law". This purported to enrol tobacco retailers into a programme of vigilance and community education about smoking being an "adult custom". Wary bureaucratic advisers to the government contacted me and asked my opinion. Because I am in contact with others doing similar work in the United States, I was quickly able to supply the bureaucrats with a piece of research that showed that participants in the programme in the United States none the less sold cigarettes to children at rates as high or higher than non-participating stores.[30]

Learning from other campaigners

There are very few public health causes that are not being addressed by others somewhere else in your country or internationally. It is true folly not to take the full implications of this on board. The first lesson among these implications is to make contact with others who are engaging in the same advocacy efforts. If you make contact with the right groups and individuals, you will potentially save yourself invaluable time, effort,

198

expense, and advocacy damage by learning from them. Read the "good books", papers, and reports in your field. Ask others what these are. They will often be repositories of valuable information and perspectives.

Letters to the editor

Although letters to the editor do not carry the implied weight of authority and expertise that editorials or opinion pieces do (*see* Editorials; Opinion page access), they are one of the most read sections of newspapers, especially in quality newspapers where the competition to get a letter published often results in a high standard of writing. Most newspapers employ staff who do nothing else but receive, read, select, edit, and verify the bona fides of letter writers whose letters are shortlisted. Apart from smaller, regional newspapers it is seldom that the actual editor of a major newspaper will read or select letters for publication.

Most letters page editors will select one or two longer letters to publish as lead letters on the top of the page. Often these will be complemented with one or two smaller letters on the same subject. Letters editors I have spoken with have shared common views about the nature of a letters page. Most were emphatic that the letters page was first and foremost a vehicle for readers and "ordinary citizens" to express their views on topical matters. They took the view that advocacy groups, politicians, government departments, and businesses were able to express their views in newspapers through the news pages or through paid advocacy advertising. Preference is therefore given to people who might express the same views as a lobby group, but who are writing as ordinary citizens.

This is not to say that letters pages will not publish letters from groups known to have a recognised position, only that to succeed, such letters often have to be quite exceptionally better than those sent in by ordinary citizens. The main exception to this rule is where a letter represents a reply or rejoinder to a previous letter which attacked or misrepresented your group or cause.

Major newspapers can receive hundreds of letters each day. When there is an important or emotive news story, the number of letters can quadruple. Yet regardless of the number of letters received, it is rare for the letters page to be expanded. There is little that is random in the fate of a letter.

A fundamental first step when attempting to have a letter published is to find out the newspaper's policy for letters to the editor. Many newspapers publish this information next to the letters they print. If it is not there, simply call the newspaper and ask in what form they would like the letter (many papers require that letters be typed, for example), and what length guidelines apply. I have never heard of a newspaper having a policy of refusing to consider faxed letters, but if in doubt, check.

Here are a few steps that will improve your chances of getting your letter printed and of making the impact you want to make.

- Be concise. Even if the paper you are writing to does not explicitly limit the length of letters it publishes, it will still be to your advantage to be as concise as possible. This rule applies to anyone who writes for a newspaper—editorialists, news reporters, columnists. With letters, the demands of brevity are even more critical.
- Stick to one angle or issue. This will help discipline the length of your letter.
- Be timely. Newspapers will rarely print issues about subjects that are not in the news. Use a current news event or recently published article as a hook for making your letter timely. Decisions about the letters for the next day's edition are often made by mid-afternoon, so if the issue you are writing about is very topical, get your letter written and delivered quickly. If you can send a letter by fax, do so.
- Keep in mind that, although you are writing for the readers of the paper, before that you are writing for one person: the letters page editor. If you don't get past this person . . . end of story. Accordingly, it is a good idea to be familiar with the different styles and genres of letters that appear on a particular paper's letters page. Are they often whimsical? Literary? Ironic? Polemical? Colloquial or formal? Is there an apparent preference for wit or metaphorical language? These sorts of questions can be helpful in shaping your approach.
- Don't assume readers will know what you are writing about. If you are writing about pending legislation, explain (briefly)

Case study: letters to editors

In late 1993, Australia's peak medical standards council, the National Health and Medical Research Council, called for the banning of professional boxing because of its propensity to cause brain damage in its participants. I wrote the following letter to the *Sydney Morning Herald*.

Several weeks ago the National Health and Medical Research Council called for professional boxing to be banned because of the brain damage it causes nearly all participants. This well-motivated but unrealistic proposal seems to have disappeared without trace. Might I suggest instead that the NH&MRC in a spirit of compromise, lobbies for the rules of boxing to be reversed? The main objective under the present rules is to hit your opponent's head so hard that his brain sloshes with such force against the skull that unconsciousness occurs. By contrast, a foul stroke is recorded when the boxer hits his opponent in the testicles. This can be very painful, occasionally dangerous, but never life-threatening. Under the reversed rules, a foul stroke would become one that strikes the head and the crowd-pleaser redefined as a lusty blow flush to the orchestra stalls [Australian rhyming slang for balls (testicles)]. Think of the new impetus to the development of evasive footwork. Think of new generations of young men with bruised egos but intact brains. With the search on for new demonstration sports for the 2000 Olympics, "cod-walloping" could be Australia's responsible entry! (*Sydney Morning Herald*, 11 December 1993)

My guess is that this letter was published because it was brief, topical, ironic, colloquial, humorous, and yet addressed a serious issue.

what that legislation is, what its effects will be, and when it will be decided. If you are writing in response to an article, editorial, or previous letter, start your letter by saying which article you are responding to (refer to the headline or writer's name) and when it appeared.
• Use your credentials. If you have personal experience or

expertise in the subject area, mention it briefly ("As someone who has had a child killed by a drunken driver . . .", "I work as a nurse in a burns ward of a large hospital . . ."). This will not only increase your chances of getting published, but it will also enhance your credibility.

- Be consistent, but original. If your organisation is planning a letter writing campaign, make sure everyone knows the facts of the situation—nothing could be worse than two letters, ostensibly on the same side of the issue, that contradict each other. At the same time, do not send in "form letters", or letters that are clearly part of a write-in campaign. No newspaper will knowingly allow itself to be part of an organisation's propaganda efforts.

- Concentrate on the local angle. Newspapers are community based organs and the letters to the editor column is where they interact with the community most explicitly. Any local angle on the subject you are writing about (how national legislation will affect a local senior citizen's centre, for example) will increase the impact of your letter and increase its chances for publication.

- Be literate. Even with serious subjects, there is no need for letters to be totally dull and earnest. Obviously your spelling and grammar should be correct but try also to write with a little flourish. Metaphors, similes, satire, literary allusions, oxymoron, and, most importantly, wit will make your letter more attractive to the letters editor and enhance its chances of being published. The letters editor of the *Sydney Morning Herald* counselled potential writers in August 1993 "The elements I miss in the letters these days are wit and whimsy. A year ago they were still present but either hard times or a trend toward political correctness, or a combination of both, is killing those delightful qualities."[31]

Two strategies are worth considering in trying to get letters published. Firstly, consider trying to get an authoritative letter published by an expert on the subject or by a well known community member. Often such people will be glad to have a letter you write go out under their signature. Secondly, try to flood the newspaper with letters from members of the community in an effort to represent widespread public opinion. If several different perspectives occur to you about how an issue might be treated in a letter, write separate letters using each approach and then quickly spread them around your coalition members or supporters for them to sign and send in. Obviously take care not to have them all typed up using the same typeface: this could alert letters editors to the letters being less "spontaneous" than they otherwise might appear.

Below are a series of letters all penned by me which were sent to an Australian news magazine signed by three different people. I sent the letters following the publication of an article that profiled an advertising agency director, Mr John Singleton, aggressively justifying his reasons for accepting a large account from the Tobacco Institute of Australia. One of the letters—the third—was published (*The Bulletin*, 15 October 1991).

Good on you John Singleton for speaking up for the tobacco farmers! I'm a smash repairer and I'd make the same points about the do-gooders who have ruined my business by reducing the road toll. Who thought about us and our families when they decided to tighten up on drunk drivers? (signed)

Here's a tip for John Singleton with his campaign to take the heat off smokers. Supposing these health fanatics are right and smoking does kill people 10 years early. Why not point this out to the government John? But in doing so, point out to them that encouraging more smoking could do much to reduce our social welfare payments and public hospital costs. By dying at say 60, smokers avoid going on the aged pension for maybe another 20 years and all the medical costs that old people run up. Our economy would be much healthier without the burden of the elderly. (signed)

John Singleton asks who worries about the tobacco farmers and their families. Let me add some others to the list: surgeons, oncologists, and undertakers. Seriously, what's going to happen to all the lung cancer specialists if smoking continues to go down? More mysteriously, why aren't they rushing to join John in his efforts? Maybe they feel there's more to life than the "right" to spend millions of dollars to convince people that carcinogenic products should be better thought of as mild, fresh and luxury length. Freedom of speech is not the same as freedom of commercial speech. (signed)

My great grandfather made a fortune selling slaves from West Africa last century, and successive generations of his family have lived in comfort as a result of his enterprise. Whatever might be thought about that sort of commerce in these so-called enlightened days, I would point out that slave trading was perfectly legal then in much the same way that smoking thankfully remains today. Should my ancestor be condemned for doing what was perfectly legal? John Singleton has my vote as a great example of a man who doesn't let namby-pamby values like preventing disease stand in the way of the right to do whatever he wants to do provided it's legal. (signed)

Letters to politicians

There is a widespread and naive view that a penultimate step in getting a law changed or a policy implemented, is simply to write to the politician in charge. This view has it that if one's concerns reflect some sensible suggestion, perhaps drawing attention to some inconsistency in policy, and are expressed soundly, the politician will put the cogs into gear and the desired changes will be set in motion. The view is naive in all sorts of ways, not the least being the assumption that your suggestion will be found in any way new or original. Most recommendations for change in major public health issues are verses from litanies that have been sung for many years.

Many politicians rarely read incoming letters personally unless they are specially passed to them by staff as being in some way important. Neither do they write their own outgoing replies, especially when it concerns routine matters such as points of view from members of the public on topical matters. Instead, bureaucratic advisers usually draft replies for the politician's signature. Often replies will be lifted out of a word processing system, containing throw away paragraphs such as "I have received many letters from constituents on the subject of the road toll. The government's view on the changes you suggest is that . . . Your views have been noted."

There are, however, ways that letter writing can help to make waves. Below are some suggestions that may enhance the chances of a politician reading, showing concern about, and perhaps even acting on the contents of letters.

How can you make the politician look good?

Change frequently involves conflict and opposition. Moves to make crash helmets compulsory for motorcyclists, for example, will bring a politician into headlong conflict with outspoken sections of the motorcycling community. Every astute politician will be fully aware of the strength of the opposition to introducing any effective measures. The decision to implement any tough public health policy will not be taken lightly, and will be balanced against the likely political gains to be made by doing so. Letters to politicians can hint at the likely reception a stand against a public health problem will have ("An epoch-making decision for community health" . . . "A principled decision in times of political spinelessness", and so on). If you have members who represent large constituencies themselves, point this out to the politician. Always write and congratulate politicians when any worthwhile action is taken so they do not feel they have acted for nothing.

Volume is important

A trickle of letters can always be dismissed by a politician as unrepresentative, especially if over the months they seem to be coming from the same handful of people. A constant stream of letters, and great rushes in response to particular incidents, can often be taken much more seriously. The tobacco industry knows the importance of keeping the letters pouring in: tobacco industry workers have been known to write letters of complaint in response to smoking control announcements. The ones I have seen, however, fell into the form letter basket (see below) and so are readily dismissed.

Don't send form letters

Form letters are standard, preprinted letters designed to be signed by your supporters and sent to politicians and other community influentials. They are meant to send a signal that there is widespread community concern about an issue. Although form letters are commonly used by advocacy groups, there is almost universal consensus among politicians that, as with most petitions (*see* Petitions), they are very ineffective means of communicating that those who send the letters actually care much about the issue. It takes little effort or commitment to sign your name on a letter you may not have even read. Politicians receive many examples of such letters and I have never heard a politician express anything but annoyance at the way they clutter up the office and require equally meaningless letters of acknowledgement to be sent to all who write.

The most inept example of this I have seen was a boxful of the same letter clearly written by management of a local tobacco factory in Sydney, signed by corralled production line workers, and sent into the New South Wales Health Minister. His office staff simply put them all in one corner and had the most junior member of the office prepare one sentence acknowledgement letters which were then stamped with an office official's signature. The effect of the letters was simply to annoy the Minister, his staff, and to add to the contempt he already held for those on the industry's side of the issue.

Although there may be total agreement about the wording of the ideal letter on a public health subject, never distribute such letters as form letters for people to either sign or retype and send. A form letter will get a form reply and nothing will be accomplished other than to affirm to the politician that your group has no imagination or political acumen. It is even risky to distribute a form listing "essential points" to be made in letters. This may result in a flood of obvious paraphrases being sent, which will leave a similar poor impression.

It is best to produce a fact sheet for distribution to potential letter writers. The sheet should provide all factual material germane to the issue you hope to have people write about, as well as summaries of the various arguments and possible responses that writers can either raise or anticipate.

Who actually writes the politician's replies?

Do some detective work and find out the name of the bureaucrat who deals with all correspondence relevant to your issue. There is a good chance that the person will be in this role because of their knowledge or background in public health and therefore possibly positively disposed to your concerns. Ask this person frankly what the politician's attitudes and positions are on the various aspects of public health policy—whether she or he is under instructions from the political party or cabinet to take a particular line, whether she or he has any personal convictions, positive or negative, about your issue, and, most importantly, whether there are any issues that the bureaucrat feels are ripe for the politician to take action on.

Letters from the powerful, the important, and the well known

Letters from persons in positions of power and influence or from public celebrities almost by definition carry more weight than those from 'ordinary' citizens. Professors, deans, heads of medical colleges, public interest groups with large memberships, trade unions, Nobel laureates, folk heroes, and bodies representing children's interests all qualify here. Even more impressive will be if several such people—say, the deans of all medical schools in the country—jointly sign a letter to a politician (*see also* Open letters).

Send copies of your letters to influential people

It may be prudent to send copies of your letters to politicians to other influential groups such as journalists, key organisations or the political opposition party. You should indicate that you have done this at the foot of your letter. If the politician feels that your letter and his or her response is being read or anticipated not only by you, but by influential people in the community, they may consider your letter more urgently and seriously.

Consider publishing your correspondence

Even if you have no immediate plans to do so, it cannot hurt your efforts to explain in your letters to politicians that you are seeking information on his or her policies for a forthcoming article, report, or book. This will help you obtain a serious and carefully worded reply, rather than some throw away line that may later embarrass its signatory. Such a prompt may even cause some reconsideration of policy, if the present policy looks archaic in the face of new information or the policies of other states or

207

nations. Care should be taken not to word such letters in belligerent terms or tones. Careful thought can produce letters that are uncompromising and to the point while not sounding hot-headed and "emotional". Always send copies of your correspondence and replies received to other groups in your network.

Litmus testing

The litmus test of whether a public health advocacy initiative is worthwhile will be your opposition's response to it. If they try to oppose an action, you're on the right track. If there is a deafening silence, you need hardly bother. The tobacco, alcohol, and junk food industries, for example, make very loud noises indeed when legislation is being proposed but seldom rustle when education is being discussed. Indeed the tobacco industry has often advocated health education as the "proper" sort of government response in the heat of its protests about impending legislative controls: John Dollison, former head of the Tobacco Institute of Australia, was reported as saying, "The industry wholeheartedly supported any sensible campaign to discourage school children from smoking"[32] and a Rothmans' spokesman wrote of "fully supporting sensible and effective public education."[33]

The message here is that you should do some quick stocktaking if your opposition remains quiet or, more worrying, supports one of your initiatives. In some circumstances you may have uncovered a "win–win" situation that benefits both your and your opposition's cause, but often your opposition may well be one step ahead of you in sensing the impact on the "big picture" goals that they are pursuing.

Local newspapers

Many advocates are dismissive of local suburban or small town newspapers because they feel that they are parochial, are simply advertising rags with a few local interest stories thrown in, have comparatively low circulations, and seldom, if ever, deal with issues likely to be compatible with significant public health advocacy. Before you are dismissive of a local newspaper as a vehicle for public health advocacy, take the time to find out if your prejudices are justified. Often they will not be. Find out the circulation and whether anything is known about its readership. Find out whether the paper is at all interested in covering stories about public health and whether it has ever taken up the cudgels for a local cause. Think about how you might localise a state or national issue for a local area readership (*see* Localisation *under* Creative epidemiology).

Young and ambitious editors and journalists working on local newspapers often nurture hopes that they can break a big story which will be picked up by a state or national news medium. If you sense that a local journalist has a sense of destiny and will "work" a local story into a state or national focus, give consideration to whether you might try to break the story locally first.

Mailing lists

Their mailing list

Your opposition may be gathering names for databases that it can call on to enlist support for its legislative proposals or in lobbying against yours. The tobacco industry, for example, has developed huge mailing lists from various give away or coupon marketing schemes.[37] You should try to get on such mailing lists so that you can know what they are up to and when. If you are well known to them, they will not be willing to put you on mailing lists. You can, however, arrange to receive their material by other means. Telephone their office in the guise of being a supporter and ask if they can send you any materials or information they have about the issues involved. Another route onto mailing lists includes any petition you may be asked to sign. Although the thought may be obnoxious, consider sending a small donation to your opposition—this will signal your support and may put you on to their mailing list extremely fast. If you attend any of their meetings incognito, often an attendance list will be passed around for people to sign. This may get you on to mailing lists, or you may be telephoned with an invitation to participate in some action that you would want to know about.

You may need to give some thought to the need to safeguard your privacy when handing out your address: tactics here include giving post office box numbers, or other people's addresses where an arrangement can be made for you to collect mail. It can be interesting to use a range of different names. This will allow you to track which avenues led your "name" to be handed to which particular database.

If all this seems somewhat devious, be assured that your opposition is getting information about you in exactly the same sorts of ways (*see* Infiltration). The first rule of politics is to *be there*: if your opposition is cooking something up and you need to know about it, a certain degree of inventiveness and cunning is often required.

Your mailing list

If your group's mailouts say nothing important, then your opposition will not be bothered to get hold of them (and perhaps you should question the effort and expense of distributing such material! Far too many public health advocacy groups tie up much of their time and effort into producing newsletters that, by the time they come out, typically describe happenings that are old news to everyone who is in any way active in the issue). Assuming that they do contain important information about strategy or tactics, then if your opposition respects you and are at all resourceful, they will try to get on your mailing list too. This means that you should exercise some care in opening up your mailing list to just anyone. In soliciting membership or supporters, you may wish to think about ways of checking just who is joining. One way of doing this is to require all who join to go through some form of scrutiny. You can explain the need for this to people so that they do not see your questions or procedures as too intrusive. Scrutiny could take the form of having joining members being recommended or nominated by existing, known, and trusted members; and being unwilling to accept post box addresses from any member not well known to your group (this will allow you to check a "doubtful" name against the addresses given using a telephone directory—if there is no listing of the name given, you may have some cause to be suspicious).

It has been my experience with the tobacco industry of

discovering that they attempt to have an employee try to attend your meeting by using his or her name and private, residential address. They also use this tactic in writing letters to the press, in the attempt to show that "ordinary citizens" share their views. If you have someone on your list who appears to be using a bona fide name and address (as checked out via the telephone directory), but whom you suspect may be an opposition plant, simply call up the head office of your opposition and say "Can I speak to [name of the suspected plant] please?" If the operator replies, "Certainly, hold the line" you will have your answer.

Mailing costs can often be a major drain on the finances of small advocacy groups. If you have many supporters who all work in the one institution—for example, a university, it will often be possible to have one of them distribute the mail to their colleagues via the institutional internal mail systems.

Marginal seats

Marginal seats are those electoral areas where a politician has only narrowly won or lost the previous political contest. In some situations, a political seat will be won or lost by literally a dozen or so votes. And where governments are elected with only the narrowest of political margins, that is, majorities of one or two seats, the importance of influencing a mere handful of voters in a marginal electorate to support your policies can take on national significance. In such situations, marginal seats are the political threads on which the life or death of whole governments and opposition parties hang.

This means that marginal seats will be inordinately interesting to political leaders particularly in the months and weeks preceding elections. If voters in these seats can be shown to be actively interested in your public health issue, it will be a foolish local politician who will ignore this interest. Reports about local support for your issue to the central policy forums of political parties by politicians in marginal seats have the capacity to transform a marginal issue into a high profile concern. Accordingly, marginal seats are frequently the scenes of intense efforts to influence voters about both political parties and single issues. Your opposition will appreciate this too and it is likely that

211

particular electorates within countries will be the focus of their efforts. If they succeed in gaining wide support for their cause in a marginal seat, irreparable damage can be done to your cause.

All public health advocates should be thoroughly familiar with which political seats in their country are marginal. Efforts should then be made to foster supportive networks within each of these areas (*see* Networks). Mailing and contact lists of groups such as doctors, churches, and community groups should be compiled and computerised. Familiarity should be developed with the local media (reporters' names, copy deadlines, and so on). This is the sort of activity that should be undertaken routinely, as part of the background preparation for advocacy work. Key opinion leaders in the area should be noted and efforts made to determine whether or not they are sympathetic to your issue. If they are, or look like they may be amenable to influence, they should be supplied with information, flattered by visits from any important campaign emissaries, and given supportive publicity via your own media access opportunities. The opposite course of action should be taken with local politicians who oppose your cause.

If your organisation is bound by its constitution or rules to be non-party political, a traditional tactic in these contexts is for lobby groups to write letters to each politician in an electorate and invite them to state their views on particular questions. Their responses, including refusals or "no comments", can then be published in advertising or on leaflets and posters. Politicians advised about the public fate of their answers will think very carefully before replying.

Media cannibalism (how media feed off themselves)

In any newspaper or broadcast news bulletin, there will be some stories that are breaking for the first time, and others that are extensions of stories which have broken earlier in other media. So in an important way, part of the definition of news is the circular statement that much news is what has already been determined to be news. (Some have even suggested that a lot of news in fact should be called "olds".) In practice this means that if one news agency decides that an issue is newsworthy, it will often be the case that its direct competitors and other forms of media will also conclude that the issue is newsworthy, even if they may have independently decided otherwise beforehand. Radio journalists seeking to fill breakfast and morning radio news programmes, for example, tend to use many of the stories that are printed in that morning's newspapers as their primary source, although naturally they will be keen to break stories that have come to light after the print media stories have gone to press. Radio journalists obtain the newspapers in the early hours of the morning while the public are asleep. A story defined as major by that morning's print media will be very compelling to radio journalists.

Similarly, any major story that has been broken by radio or daytime television will be picked up by evening television and by print journalists writing their stories for the next morning's edition. Journalists who are covering a story that has already been broken in another medium will be seeking to extend the story in a way that makes it look like they are not simply repeating others' material. In these ways, the media are constantly cannibalising their fellow outlets.

For public health advocates, this means that they must think of news opportunities in two ways. Besides trying to interest the news media in original stories, they must place themselves in the position of journalists and be constantly anticipating ways in which to assist journalists in *extending* stories. Most successful public health advocates are avid news addicts: they get up early to read newspapers, they wake to radio news bulletins, have news programmes on in the car and watch news and current affairs programmes as much as they can.

Media conferences

Media conferences are one of the standard vehicles in any advocate's stable of strategies. Media conferences are essentially meetings where the media are invited *en masse* for a specific purpose. These purposes can include:

- Releasing statements and providing detailed commentary.
- The launch of something new (books, reports, products, services).

● An opportunity to interview a celebrity or authority.

A media conference should be held whenever you anticipate that the story you have is likely to be of interest to a wide range of the media. In holding a conference you are saying to the media that your story is big enough to invite representatives from many different newspapers, radio, and television. It is also important to put yourself in the shoes of the media and ask whether there is any perceived advantage to them in covering your story face to face at a news conference, or whether it could just as adequately be covered by a journalist telephoning you. If you conclude that the conference does not have obvious allure, then you will need to put thought into making it more tantalising.

Journalists regularly try to ascertain whether other media (and particularly their rivals) will be covering a story or attending a media conference. A missed story, particularly a big one, is considered very bad form in journalistic circles. So if you have the assurance from particular journalists that they will be attending your conference, it is a good idea to spread such information to other media in a passing mention.

The timing and place of media conferences are important. You should become familiar with the schedules and deadlines of the programmes or editions in which you want to have your story covered and hold the conference at a time which will allow the journalists to attend, write or edit their story, and allow for any other commitments that may be in their schedules. In planning the day for the conference, you should try to anticipate any competition from other stories (*see* Slow news days) and consider that journalists will need to buy their lunch (so if you provide it, you may well tip the scales more towards their attendance!).

When you hold media conferences, advantage should be taken of any venues that will be a poignant reminder of the more dramatic aspects of your public health issue. Rooms adjacent to cancer wards, forensic medicine, or post-mortem lecture theatres (which are often located near morgues) or general hospital locations are ideal. Someone active in your field will probably be connected with such a venue, and so holding a meeting there will not appear contrived or melodramatic.

In such locations, a major prong of your opposition's position —that the health consequences of (for example) smoking or drink

214

driving are the exaggerated fabrications of fanatics—will be rendered an objection in the poorest possible taste.

Checklist for media conferences*

- Have the date, time and place been cleared with all speakers?
- Are the time and place suitable for the reporters from media you are most concerned to attract to the event or media conference?
- Are there any predictable media conflicts (other major events or media conferences) that you know about?
- Is the room large enough?
- Are there telephones nearby and plenty of electrical outlets for television lights?
- Will you need a public address system?
- Have people been assigned to clean up the room before and after the conference?
- Do you plan to serve refreshments? Has this been arranged?
- Who is sending out the media releases?
- Have you checked to see that the fax numbers for the releases are still current?
- Who is making follow up calls to editors and reporters? Are these people properly briefed about the event and the issue?
- Are visuals, charts, etc required for the media conference?
- Does each speaker know what the other speakers are going to say?
- Is someone drafting a question and answer sheet for anticipated questions at the media conference?
- Has provision been made for all speakers to rehearse their presentations and answers to the anticipated questions?
- Are materials being prepared for a media kit or a media release?

---

* Adapted from Bobo K, Kendall J, Max S. *Organize! Organizing for social change. A manual for activists in the 1990s*. Washington: Seven Locks Press, 1991:123.

215

Media etiquette

Like any group of professionals, journalists have standard operating procedures that should be respected by anyone who chooses to interact with them. The following are some tips you should always keep in mind:

- Respect deadlines. Whenever you talk with any journalist about a story, first ask them if they are on a deadline. If they are, respect it. One of the quickest ways to lose a journalist's respect is to call them with help on a story after the deadline has passed.
- Don't consider reporters to be your friends (or your enemies). After they have developed a friendly relationship with a journalist, many advocates are tempted to ask the journalist to "join the cause". Many journalists make it plain to you, off the record, that they have a great deal of sympathy with your cause. There is a huge difference, however, between them expressing this to you personally and their wishing to do anything more than report your story. Attempting to cross such a boundary may be embarrassing for the journalist who may avoid subsequent contact with you. It is hard for some advocates to realise that journalists who frequently write favourable stories are not their allies. A journalist's job is to write about an issue, not to help you in your cause. This should be respected. Equally, journalists who write unfavourable stories are not necessarily your enemies. Agree to disagree with them. After all, they may see your side one day.
- Follow up on promises. If journalists ask for information you don't have and you promise to provide it later, do so. Journalists depend on their sources; if you do not follow up on your promises you are not only making it difficult for them to do their job, you may seriously damage your credibility as a source.
- Don't be petty. If journalists fail to use your quote, or fail to give your organisation prominent enough mention, do not act as if they have failed to do their job. Keep the big picture in mind. This applies especially to the common practice of minor misquotation. Journalists will sometimes paraphrase what you have said to them, with the result that expressions or

emphases are used which are not exactly the way you would have preferred to see a report appear. In such cases, it is wise to consider the impact on the journalist of any complaint you might make. It is preferable to be seen by journalists as a good and reliable source, than as a sensitive pedant who has to be treated with kid gloves.

I was recently quoted in an Australian newspaper as saying, "If reformed gun laws saved even one life, they would be worthwhile." This is a clichéd media expression that I know I never use, and while I found it irritating to read such cant attributed to me, the overall tenor of the article was positive. To have complained to the journalist or her editor would have probably meant she would be reluctant to contact me next time the gun issue came up—clearly a poor advocacy outcome.

Media logs

Most radio and television stations keep a record or log of calls from the public who call up to praise, complain, or otherwise comment on programmes. Sometimes callers are switched through to an answering machine; others summarise calls into a log book. Many lobbies arrange for their members and supporters to inundate such programmes with calls. In Australia, for example, the pro-gun and anti-abortion lobbies both swamp the switchboards of programmes who run items featuring spokespeople whom these lobbies oppose. Often the inundation is so obviously orchestrated that it is not taken seriously as a sign of community feeling. However, the programme logs are set up because journalists and media management are keenly interested in taking the pulse of audiences in as many ways as possible. Encouraging your supporters to telephone in their praise or criticism can thus be an important way of sending messages to key influentials in the media.

Some programmes do not seem to mind allowing you access to their logs, especially if you have been of assistance to them in making the programme or have appeared in it. Such access can provide some interesting insights into how the public reacted to you or your opposition.

Media releases

A media release (often known as a press release) is simply a means of sending a statement to the media with the intention that it will inspire the issues contained in it to become news. If a media release achieves its purpose, it will almost invariably cause the media to contact the author or contact person listed on it. This means that you should be prepared to take matters further than they have been expressed in the release, which means that you should prepare some notes to prompt you when journalists begin to phone for interviews.

The checklist below lists some of the more important points to attend to in composing a media release. Some people baulk at the idea of putting their private telephone numbers on a media release, fearing invasion of privacy or even security problems. On the other hand, 24 hour contact is extremely important to the success of a media release. You must appreciate that the media do not work to a nine to five schedule, and that, if they cannot reach you to check a story or conduct an interview, the story will often die and the whole point of putting out the release will be lost.

If you have strong privacy or security concerns, the only options are to use others as spokespeople who do not share these concerns, or else to use a diversion telephone (where the number listed on the release is not your home number, but is programmed to divert your call to your home, unbeknown to those who are calling you). A paging service (where callers are put through to a paging service who then notify you through a paging device to call back those who have telephoned) is also an option, although usually an expensive one.

Checklist for media releases*

- Is the release on organisational letterhead?
- Is the release dated and marked for immediate release or embargoed until a specific day and time?
- Is the contact person's name and phone number (day and evening) listed at the top of the release?
- Is the headline short and pithy? Is it arresting, relevant, and succinct?
- Is the copy double spaced?
- Does the first paragraph explain who, what, why, when, and where?
- Have you quoted key individuals in the second and third paragraphs? Have you cleared the quotes with them first?
- Is each page marked with an abbreviated headline? (Try to keep the release to two pages—one is better—two can become separated on a journalist's desk and rendered useless.)
- Is a photo opportunity mentioned if there is one? If so, also send the release to the photo editor.

Networks and coalitions

In advocacy work, "networks" are generally informal webs of loosely affiliated groups and individuals who share common concerns. Regardless of your cause, it is important to identify and make contact with other groups which might lend numbers, power, resources, prestige, an inviolate credibility, or some unique association to your public health initiatives. There exist formidable networks such as medical associations and societies, the consumer movement, trade unions, parent groups, churches, victim groups, and international networks of issue specific activists whose experience and contacts can prove invaluable to advocacy work.

Coalitions are more defined groupings of different interest

* Adapted from Bobo K, Kendall J, Max S. *Organize! Organizing for social change. A manual for activists in the 1990s.* Washington: Seven Locks Press, 1991:123.

groups which join forces around particular issues or specific tasks (for example, to lobby for a particular piece of legislation or in protest against a particular policy). There are enormous advantages, and occasionally disadvantages, to be gained from forming a coalition. Individual groups within coalitions will often have their own publicity and information distribution networks through which your issue can be publicised.

It is important to have all coalition members make specific personal, financial, and institutional commitments to any advocacy initiative with which their name is associated.[35-37] When you invite any group to join a coalition, you should take time to determine the degree of commitment that you might expect from the new group. Many coalitions have members who are merely passengers—dead weights to the efforts of others who use up valuable resources insisting on being kept informed and so on, but never really contributing. Early clarity about a group's involvement will benefit all concerned.

Computer networking

A crucial element of media advocacy is information—information about your issue, your opposition, and the efforts of your colleagues. Timely information not only alerts you to media advocacy opportunities but can also help you learn about and from the media advocacy activities of others. Information can be gleaned from a variety of sources including newsletters, conferences, regular telephone calls to other advocates, industry trade magazines, etc. One new method of sharing a lot of information quickly and efficiently is through computer networks. Computer networks link advocates on specific issues together via their personal computers and modems. Computer networks exist for the arms control, abortion rights, and smoking control communities, among others.

Open letters

Private letters to politicians run the risk of achieving nothing but a polite reply, with no one but staff knowing the extent and vehemence of community feeling towards your public health issue. Public or open letters are read by thousands, and millions in some countries. You should weigh up what effects you hope to achieve—gentle, polite persuasion or public confrontation—before deciding to write privately or publicly, as described below. An open letter is a letter to a particular individual such as a politician, the managing director of an industry that is affecting public health, or a sporting hero who helps in tobacco promotions, and which is published in a newspaper. Open letters should always ask direct questions which allow those to whom they are addressed no latitude in evading answers. Open letters are the advocate's equivalent of politicians' parliamentary questions to their political opposition. Like parliamentary questions, open letters are on the public record, cannot easily be avoided, and allow the public to "eavesdrop" on a personal exchange about matters of public importance.

If your issue is one that is of public significance, the person "receiving" the open letter will hardly be able to avoid answering the questions asked, because any silence on his or her part is likely to be subject to inquiries from journalists. In other words, the open letter and its sequelae may well become news in itself.

Open letters are occasionally accepted as letters to the editor ("Having written on many occasions to [name of politician etc] and received evasive replies, I would like to ask [politician X] through your newspaper to answer the following questions: . . ."). Open letters may also be placed in a press release, with the hope that the text of the full letter will be published in news reports based on the release. If you use this option, the letter should be sent directly to the person to whom it is addressed as well, so that your press release can describe how the letter has been sent, the background to its sending and so on. This course of action risks failure if few or no news media pick up your press release.

The most direct way of publishing open letters is to run them as a paid advertisement. This may not be possible if your organisation has too low a budget. Fundraising or celebrity funding (see Advertising in advocacy) may make this possible.

Elizabeth Whelan of the American Council on Science and Health has regularly written to the US Tobacco Institute asking blunt questions about matters such as what product safety criteria the industry uses in formulating its products. She never receives answers to her questions but publishes her letters and the Institute's evasive replies in the Council's newsletter.

Opinion (op-ed) page access

Most papers publish an opinion page opposite the editorial page. This opinion page contains columns written by the paper's own columnists and syndicated columnists. In some cases, newspapers will publish guest columns or opinion pieces written by academics, experts, and public authorities.

Although many newspapers consider it a high priority to maintain open access to their opinion pages, not all papers are receptive to publishing guest pieces from non-staff, let alone special interest groups. If your paper is averse to running pieces by overt advocacy groups, you may be able to have your issue covered by having a sympathetic academic submit the piece under his or her name, which may lend the article extra "authority" in the eyes of the editors. If you want to write on behalf of your organisation, it's important to know the policy of your paper. Reading the paper regularly will also tell you the editorial direction of the paper. This is important to know, because papers will generally see no need for a guest column unless it is filling some void. No paper will want to print a guest column that is merely echoing what another columnist has already written or what has already been articulated by the paper in an editorial. In fact, your best bet may be to write an article that takes a contrary position to an editorial.

When you've decided what you want to write, telephone or arrange a meeting with the opinion page editor to discuss your ideas. Tell him or her if you want to write in response to something that has been printed in the paper or if you want to express your views on a subject. Whenever someone in your group delivers a speech, writes a column for a newsletter, or writes a summary of a report or study, consider whether or not that might be a good basis for a guest column in the paper.

If your idea is accepted by the paper, find out how long they would like the piece to be, and when they need it. When you know the deadline, observe it. There is no quicker way to ruin your credibility with a newspaper than by not respecting their time restrictions. No newspaper will accept anything sight unseen, and all advocates have known the frustrations and disappointment of being given the green light to submit a piece, only never to have it printed.

Start by outlining what you want to write—not only the issue but the point of view you want to take as well. Consider what the paper has already printed on the subject and decide how you could best contribute to the debate. Above all, be sensitive to the needs of newspapers to publish readable, engaging material. Ask yourself, and have others tell you before you send off your contribution, whether what you have written reads well. Would an ordinary reader who was inexpert or not close to the issue find it meaningful and interesting? Are you using bureaucratic or ghetto language (see Jargon and ghetto language)? Do you make assumptions of the reader's knowledge that are unreasonable?

Opinion polls

Opinion polls on your issue, particularly those conducted in marginal seats (see Marginal seats) or adjacent to elections are a time honoured advocacy strategy. Favourable results from polls can be used to assure politicians that there is strong community support for your issue, and that any suggestion that your concerns are fringe or unrepresentative are unwarranted. Results from polls can also be useful as a focal point for media releases.

Commercial opinion poll organisations are polling the community for their clients all year round. They have infrastructures to deal with question design, sampling, interviewing (door to door or telephone), collation and analysis of results, and reporting that are often highly efficient and frequently of a standard that will pass most tests of methodological acceptability. Many of these companies conduct "omnibus" surveys where they present a string of questions commissioned by different clients to samples of the population. The cost of having one or several questions added to these omnibus surveys can often be surprisingly affordable even to groups with modest budgets. If the cost is out of reach, consider pooling resources with some other members of your network to buy a few questions.

Case study: opinion polls

Cricket in Australia has long received huge sums from the Benson and Hedges tobacco company. When a politician tried to have a bill introduced to ban tobacco sponsorship of sport, an Australian cricketing association advertised that it had set up a public opinion voting phone line. The public were invited to phone and register their support or opposition to the proposed bill. Callers to the line who wanted to register their support for the ban were told that only opposing calls were being recorded. Two days later, the Tobacco Institute of Australia published a large press advertisement where results of a "cricket poll" were stated as "90% opposed, 10% in favour" of the ban. The realities of the fabricated "poll" were then given high profile exposure on prime time television[38] and made the subject of a formal complaint to the Advertising Standards Council, which upheld the complaint.

The public has a healthy disrespect for survey results. This can work both against your own use of polls, and also for you when you attack dubious poll results being promoted by your opponents. Your opponents' polls should be subject to scrutiny for practices such as leading questions or those inducing bias, series effects (the practice of asking a key question after several others, the answers to which virtually induce respondents into producing a desired answer), inadequate samples, or lack of independence in those who conduct the poll. If you have a survey expert among your supporters, routinely subject your opposition's polls to this person for criticism.

Opportunism

A media advocacy campaign is like a political campaign in which competing forces continuously react to unexpected events, breaking news items, and opportunities, rather than conducting

---

Case study: opportunism

In the opening week of the 1993 Australian federal election, the conservative (Liberal) opposition party ran a television advertisement showing the sights of a rifle focusing on a range of different individuals. The intent of the advertisement was to draw a violent analogy between citizens being "picked off" their jobs by unemployment said to be caused by the policies of the Government. The Coalition for Gun Control put out a media release calling on the Liberal Party to withdraw the advertisement because of its gross insensitivity to its own, often stated, position on reducing violence in the community. The rifle/sniper image had been widely discussed by broadcast commentators as being "disturbing" and "perhaps inappropriate" so when the Coalition on Gun Control came into the debate, the media seized on their comments as highly newsworthy. The Opposition leader spent the better part of a valuable day of the election campaign having to respond to the gun violence issue, and the Prime Minister, smelling his Opposition's electoral blood, made many supportive comments about the terror of gun violence. The press release made the front page of the national newspaper, the *Australian*.[39]

---

a static, preformed educational campaign. For this reason, opportunism is central to the nature of effective media advocacy. To describe someone as an opportunist is generally to cast a slur on their character. In advocacy though, a nose for opportunism is, without doubt, an invaluable and indispensable trait. In fact, it is probably the single most important quality that an effective advocate can develop. There are innumerable examples in public health of quite unplanned media coups occurring through individuals having a nose for opportunities to exploit newsworthy events and issues by offering alternative angles that satisfy media appetites for "the other side". The most successful public health advocates have not taken a casual, serendipitous attitude to the search for opportunities, but actively cast about for new ways to raise public health issues onto the public agenda. There

Case study: opportunism

When William Bennett was nominated to be President Bush's first drug control "czar", an *ad hoc* coalition of smoking control groups sponsored a full page newspaper advertisement issuing Bennett a "drug free challenge" to give up his $2\frac{1}{2}$ pack a day cigarette habit. The newspaper advertisement ran in the *Washington Times* (not the much more expensive *Washington Post*) the day before the start of Bennett's Senate confirmation hearings, and was supported by a similar radio advertisement that ran a few times on a local Washington station. That small investment was enough to reach millions. The story was carried in outlets such as the *Washington Post* (which referred to the effort as a "multi-media campaign"), the *New York Times, USA Today*, and the Mutual Broadcasting Network.

Case study: opportunism

Another example of creative opportunism involved the Food and Drug Administration's ban on all fruit imports from Chile because of some tainted grapes. At the Smoking Control Advocacy Resource Centre in Washington DC, staff investigations found that the whole episode started because two grapes in Philadelphia were each found to contain 3 µg of cyanide. A quick check of information in recent US Surgeon General's reports showed that every single cigarette contains several hundred micrograms of cyanide. In fact, the sidestream smoke emitted from a single cigarette contains up to 110 µg of hydrogen cyanide, which is more potent than the sodium cyanide found in the grapes. All fruit imports from an entire country were banned because of two grapes containing a tiny fraction of only one of the poisons in cigarettes. That was news.

Case study: opportunism

Sydney activist Peter Vogel wrote to the Mercedes-Benz company on 18 April 1985, questioning whether approval had been given for their cars to be used in an advertisement for Sterling cigarettes. He suggested that associations of safety and prestige from Mercedes' reputation were being transferred to the cigarettes. Mercedes' solicitor replied "I can assure you that the ad . . . [was] published entirely without this company's participation or approval . . . This company would prefer that its products were never used by others, whether directly or indirectly, in their promotional material . . . we rely entirely upon the integrity and courtesy of the advertiser in first consulting us over the form and content of a proposed ad and then abiding by our wishes in the matter. In the present case, this was not done." Vogel's opportunist initiative may have driven a further nail into the coffin containing the tattered remnants of the industry's integrity in the business world.

---

are few guidelines that can convert you into a good opportunist other than to advise that public health advocates should be constantly assessing opportunities that can provide a "peg" for a media comment. The case studies above and following are some examples.

Parody

In 1987 the Australian Council on Smoking and Health in Perth published an "alternative" annual report for a fictitious tobacco company.[40] Produced in a luscious glossy cover, the report featured a "death yield table" where brand share of different cigarettes was apportioned into the total number of deaths caused by tobacco in Australia for that year. The report went on to explain that the directors of this fictitious tobacco company had now decided to accept the evidence on smoking and disease, and quoted approvingly a resignation speech from a former

---

Case study: parody

BUGA UP, the Australian graffiti group, regularly produced parodies of theatre, ballet, and concert programmes for events sponsored by tobacco companies. BUGA UP members, dressed in formal evening wear, would mingle in the foyers with the audiences for these events and distribute the fake programmes to the unsuspecting patrons. On opening their "programmes", they would read material, partly humorous and partly serious, about BUGA UP's position on tobacco sponsorship. The programmes asked for donations to be sent to BUGA UP and these were often received.

Chairman of Carreras Rothmans in Northern Ireland who said, "I could not quite get it [working for a tobacco company] squared with my conscience." The report was launched with all the pomp and ceremony of a real company report and attracted much media attention.

Petitions

Petitions—lists of names, addresses and signatures of people supporting your issue or demanding that a politician or authority take some action—are an age old advocacy tactic. In the United States, in about 20 states, they can be essential to the process of having referenda put to voters so that laws initiated by citizens can be enacted. In Montana, for example, petitions from 5% of registered voters are required to have a proposition placed before all voters.[35] Petitions can operate at the local neighbourhood level—for example, having residents petition local government about the need for traffic calming—in the workplace, such as petitioning management to improve canteen food, or on state and national issues.

Generally speaking, the effectiveness of petitions lies in direct proportion to the extent that they are perceived to represent a majority of citizens in a given area, coupled with the consideration of what sort of commitment is implied by someone merely going to the minor trouble of signing their name. Small neighbourhood petitions which include the signatures of most residents are likely to make their point more forcibly to a local government body than comparatively large, community-wide petitions which can be shown to be none the less unrepresentative.

The principle that a chain is only as strong as its weakest link can apply to petitions. If a petition has names on it which can be shown to be fictitious ("Mr Donald Duck" or simply names which, when verified at the address given, are shown not to exist), doubt can be cast on the whole petition. If you are aware or suspect that names on your opponents' petitions are fictitious, it can be devastating to alert the media to this. Equally, if you are in the business of collecting signatures yourself for a petition, it is wise to require all those who are signing to provide identification to the person collecting the signatures. The reason for this should be explained to those who are inconvenienced when signing.

It is also wise to put a lot of thought into how to collect a lot of signatures most efficiently. The main way to do this is to avoid time consuming methods such as door to door approaches, when opportunities exist to approach many people who gather together in places such as workplaces, shopping centres, sporting events, queues, churches, meetings, and so forth. "Snowballing" techniques for example, asking the particularly keen among those who sign to take a copy of the petition sheet and themselves collect signatures—should also be considered.

Pictures and graphics

Watch any news bulletin on television and observe what is shown. Typically each item will commence with the newsreader in camera introducing the story. As he or she reads, it is common that a still shot or graphic illustrative of the story will be on screen behind the newsreader. Very early into the news piece, the film will cut to either file film or footage recorded that day on the story being dealt with. On big, dramatic "on-the-spot" items that are occurring while the news bulletin is going to air, the cut may be to a live shot involving a reporter.

Television is an essentially visual medium and news producers are always keen to illustrate any story with an apposite and arresting scene. It is a very rare television news story that does not feature film footage in some way. Advocates can take no interest in this aspect of their news stories, or they can take steps to try and influence what is shown as the story is being read. If you don't orchestrate how your story will be illustrated, the media will do it for you, and will sometimes get things horribly wrong, giving an emphasis to the story that may distract greatly from your ideal framing.

If you are going to be interviewed or photographed for a press story, think about the location where you will ask the media to meet you. Many television journalists and editors regard the "talking head" shot of a person being interviewed or making a speech as boring television, often more likely to end up on the cutting room floor than being broadcast. Anticipate this reaction, no matter how important you feel the news value of your story might be. If you can make your talking head points in a setting which is visually relevant to the issue at hand (in front of a polluting factory; outside a school where the school canteen refuses to sell a range of healthier food for children; on the steps of the head office of your opposition; a burns ward in a hospital if your issue is unsafe flammable children's nightwear; a car wrecker's yard if your issue is drunken driving). Such settings will generally appeal to media gatekeepers more than the usual talking head shot of an expert or spokesperson in front of a shelf of books or sitting at a desk.

The media are also always thirsty for good graphical depictions of the data you are dealing with. "Good" basically means simple and readily comprehensible to viewers or readers, expressing no more than one or two relationships between variables. Have colour versions of these ready for journalists who may be keen to include them in a story.

"Piggy backing"

Riding your story on the back of a stronger one that is running a good race in the media is a time honoured media advocacy

Case study: piggy backing

In October 1990, Australia's wealthiest man, publishing billionaire Kerry Packer, suffered a heart attack. For some minutes, Packer was clinically "dead", but was revived with a cardiac defibrillator carried by the ambulance that attended him. On his recovery, Packer donated $3.5 million to the NSW State Health Department to enable defibrillators to be installed in every ambulance in NSW. His magnanimity and concern to save lives was an instant headline story and the devices have since been referred to as "Packer whackers" by ambulance teams. At the time, Packer's Australian television network carried the rights to broadcast the summer-long tobacco (Benson and Hedges) sponsored cricket. I wrote a letter to the *Sydney Morning Herald* praising Packer's generosity, but making the point that his concern to save people from deaths from heart disease would find fuller expression if he were to publicly refuse to continue to accept the tobacco sponsored cricket on his television network. The letter generated considerable debate in the media.

Case study: piggy backing

On the day that the eminent and high profile Australian eye surgeon Professor Fred Hollows died with a last wish that donations, not flowers, be sent to his memorial Foundation to help support interocular lens factories and implant programmes in Eritrea, Nepal, and Vietnam, a prominent Australian footballer was awarded $350 000 damages against a magazine that had run an unauthorised photograph which showed his penis in an after-match shower. The footballer had argued that his reputation as a role model for children was endangered by the implication that he had given permission for the photograph to be published. Supporters of the Hollows Foundation lost no time in making press comment that if the footballer was indeed sincere in his motivation, and that venal concerns were not paramount, then he would donate the awarded damages to the Foundation.

strategy. The idea is to latch on to the interest being shown by the media in a particular story and provide a new twist or angle that will enable the media to extend the life of the original story. The bigger the original story, the broader the shoulders on which your new twist story can ride. If you see that there are apposite parallels or ironies with your issue in the reporting of a news story, the media will often find this worth reporting.

Press agencies

Press agencies such as Reuters, United Press International, and Australian Associated Press are journalistic agencies which cover stories and then distribute the stories to news outlets, often worldwide, which may have been unable to cover a story first hand. These agencies can be very important in obtaining maximum coverage for your issue. They have particular value in getting coverage for local issues that may have worldwide interest, but which are not mammoth hard news stories that will have sold themselves worldwide. In public health, good examples of this are often research reports appearing in medical journals. These may not have been big enough news stories to make the front page of a national paper, but they may have been covered some way into the national press. By giving a press agency an opportunity to cover such a story, it may well be picked up around the world, which in turn can sometimes give it an extra newsworthy boost at home (*see* Media cannibalism).

Props

When you are being interviewed on television, being photographed by the press or addressing public meetings, appropriate props can often be used to good effect. Stan Glantz, an American tobacco control advocate, often found himself in debating situations with tobacco industry representatives who sought to trade blows using research reports. They would typically have dug up some obscure study that suggested tobacco was in some way not to blame for the mortality of a group of people. They would use this to frame the debate in terms of: "There is certainly not consensus about this tobacco and health issue." Anticipating

---

Case study: props

Dr Arthur Chesterfield-Evans once held a press conference on the steps of the head office of an Australian tobacco company. He wished to make some statements about the company's irresponsibility in advertising tobacco. Chesterfield-Evans obtained some blood soaked sheep lungs from his local butcher and took them to the press conference in a plastic bucket. During his press conference speech, the respectably dressed doctor plunged his immaculately cuffed hand into the bucket, drew out the lungs and talked about the surgical consequences of the actions of the marketing executives seated inside the building. Again, the prop worked to great effect in terms of media coverage.

---

this debating ploy, Glantz once took with him a computer printout that was sitting on a desk in his office. When the anticipated ploy began to be used, Glantz concertinaed the lengthy printout all over the floor of the studio, explaining that this was just a month's worth of recently published evidence further corroborating the smoking/disease nexus. He calculated that neither the interviewer nor his opponent would have time to examine the printout and fuss about details. The prop had the desired effect.

Similarly, the 1979 United States Surgeon General's report on smoking was reportedly deliberately published in an ungainly, fat doorstopper sized, single volume to reinforce dramatically the message that there was an awful lot of research on the issue. The thinking was that many advocates might have an opportunity to wave the mammoth tome in front of television cameras, powerfully reinforcing the point that they were making.

Publicising others' research

Scientific research published in medical and public health journals is regularly used as a source for news stories (*see*

Chapters 2 and 3). A recent American study found that 65% of first authors of papers published in the *Journal of the American Medical Association* or the *New England Journal of Medicine* had received some media coverage of their paper, with a majority receiving media coverage from more than one medium.[5] Some medical journals employ public relations consultants or staff to better ensure that scientific articles in their journals are covered by the media. Most do not, however, with the result that many potentially great newsworthy scientific articles are read only by a relative handful of specialists who subscribe to such specialist journals or who read them in libraries.

Public health advocates can act as the absent public relations people for such journals by simply bringing the media's attention to potentially newsworthy articles. Serious public health advocates should be able to identify all of the main specialist journals favoured by researchers in their field. They should also routinely check new issues in their nearest public health library. It may be prudent to allocate an hour or so a week as time when someone with an eye for likely newsworthiness can scan through electronic databases such as *Current Contents* for newly published papers. These can then be obtained from the authors or libraries. If the researchers are local or contactable, get in touch with them and explain that you would like to see their work given a wider audience in the media. Ask if they would be amenable to talking with the media and suggest that you could prepare a press release, have them check it for accuracy, and then you would take care of sending it out to the media.

If the researchers have had no experience with the media, demystify the likely course of events that will follow for them if the media take an interest in the story.

Quotes

It is a good idea to develop the habit of keeping a dossier of revealing statements made by your opposition. Over the years, your opposition will have made statements that they can look back on with embarrassment: statements that are contradictory, indiscreet, intended for private audiences, or simply horrendous gaffes that they wish they could forget. They will also have spoken and written often on their position in forums where they expect that only their supporters will be attentive. Here they may have written things that would be couched in more cautious terms if voiced in more public situations. Keep these on file cross referenced by the person or organisation which made them, and by subject. Such quotes can be put to dramatic effect during debates and interviews and on pamphlets and handbills.

In the 1987 campaign in the United States, to block Ronald Reagan's nomination of the arch conservative Judge Robert Bork to the US Supreme Court, a "book of Bork" was compiled which exhaustively documented 25 years of Bork's writings, speeches, and judgments on a diverse range of issues which collectively gave ample demonstration of Bork's values and politics.[41] The "book of Bork" became central in the successful campaign to defeat his nomination.

Radicalism

Many public health issues attract the interest of individuals who are impatient for change and unconstrained by having conflicts of loyalty to an employing agency's policies. Their agenda for change may share much in common with yours, but go a great deal further in both goals and strategies. Often such individuals will alarm those who are working in or near "the system". Conservative individuals will complain that those with radical goals and strategies risk alienating those with power and influence to change things; they fear that radicalism will frighten moderates away from supporting an issue.

Radical groups and ideas, however, have often been of critical importance in the process of successful public health advocacy. Perhaps the most important historical function of radicalism is the way that it can redefine as moderation that which had formerly seemed radical. Before the emergence in the early 1980s of the Australian anti-tobacco billboard graffiti group BUGA UP, the calls by establishment health and medical organisations for total bans on tobacco advertising had seemed draconian to many sections of the Australian population. BUGA UP's wit and uncompromising spray-painted criticisms gradually transformed the mild mannered positions of the establishment groups into commonplaces that were less confronting to governments not wanting to be seen to move ahead of public opinion. This resulted in a gradual drift by even conservative parties towards the centre ground, newly defined by BUGA UP's radicalism. The result was that, within a decade, the tobacco advertising ban position drew all-party support (see the introduction in Part I).

Similarly, in the United States in the 1960s, Malcolm X's civil rights radicalism, embodied in the theme "By any means necessary", led to the rise in influence of Martin Luther King. King gained access to a wide array of influential people because they preferred dealing with him than with Malcolm X.[42]

Civil disobedience

There have been many instances of civil disobedience (law breaking) in the history of public health. The work of Greenpeace in the environmental health area is perhaps the most prominent contemporary example. Civil disobedience can carry with it a Robin Hood subtext (outlaws who work for the public good) which forces the public to confront which set of values it believes to be more important. BUGA UP members, for example, were constantly vilified by the tobacco and outdoor advertising industries as being "vandals" for altering the wording on outdoor advertising posters (figure 9). BUGA UP was confident that the great majority of the public would perceive the vandalism of eyesore ephemera such as advertising hoardings to be instantly understandable as being a lesser "wrong" than the flagrant courting of new recruits into smoking.

Reporters and journalists

Reporters and journalists are the media workers with whom public health advocates deal most. It is therefore important to understand how they work, how they see their jobs, what sort of things motivate and please them, and to try generally to see their work from their perspective. If you can do this, you will be better able to develop a mutually valued relationship with journalists.

Perhaps the most important thing that should be said about

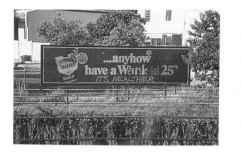

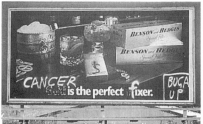

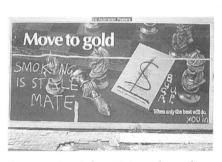

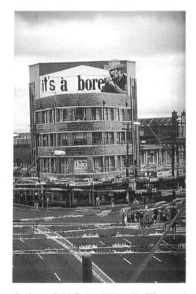

Figure 9: Advertising hoardings altered by BUGA UP (Billboard Utilising Graffitists Against Unhealthy Promotions): (top left) lending a hand at ridding smoking control of its puritan image; (top right) the original slogan read "Gold is the perfect mixer"; (bottom left) another example of civil disobedience recruited into the public health cause; (bottom right) this message was put across at one of Sydney's busiest intersections.

your relationship with reporters and journalists is that they need you just as much as you need them. Understanding this can develop mutual respect that can be rewarding for advocates and journalists alike: you will get your issues covered in the media and they will write stories which get published or broadcast, thereby helping their own career paths. If they do not know of your existence, or if they find your cause or the way you present it dull and unnewsworthy, you will have no mutually beneficial relationship. If they know and respect you as a regular news source or commentator, however, they will seek you out as someone who helps them get their job done.

The second main point to be made about journalism is that they are journalists, not public health advocates. Their job is to produce copy that will pass upward through the various editorial filters that operate in news organisations and into print or broadcasts. To fulfil this goal, their presentation of their stories has to satisfy the criteria of newsworthiness that were described in Chapters 2–4. Their job is *not* to be fifth column public health educators. If their work *in fact* is effective public education or advocacy, then there will have been a happy coincidence of advocacy and journalistic agenda. Often though, journalists will not give the emphasis to a story that you would have hoped for it. Although you may be disappointed in this, it is thoroughly inappropriate to blame journalists for somehow falling short of a mark that you as an advocate have set for their work. To act in such a way would be to wholly misunderstand what journalists are there to do (*see* Chapter 2 for a discussion of the work constraints and imperatives of journalism).

Advocates who work every day in a particular area are sometimes disappointed to discover that many in the media do not know about their expertise and dedication, or even their existence. This is true even for the advocates of well established groups. Part of the reason for this is that staff changes in news organisations can be rapid: the reporters covering various rounds like health and medicine, politics or features tend to move on to other rounds quickly, so that the reporter you dealt with next time may be quite new to the area and quite unaware of your group, the issues involved and the history of a particular debate.

Eventually, if you prove yourself to be an open, credible, dependable, and trustworthy source, you won't have to worry about attracting the media's attention because they will come looking for you. Becoming known as a good source can take time, however, so be patient.

The first step in establishing access to the media in your community is to let them know that you exist. Find out which reporters cover the issues on which you work. This may not be as obvious as it seems. Public health issues, for example, might at one time or another be covered by reporters on all of the following rounds: health; business; sport; cooking and leisure; legislation; or politics. Stories about public health might also be assigned by editors of the national, state, local, or business desks.

The best way to determine which reporters and editors are responsible for the issues that interest you is to read the paper and look at the bylines. If you're not a regular, careful reader, do some research. Most newspapers have back issues indexed by subject in their libraries and will give you access to them. The major newspapers can also be found on file at libraries.

Once you have determined which reporters you need to know, initiate contact with them. You can do this by sending them a letter that advises them of your interests and areas of expertise. Tell them you would like to be put on their files of contacts and are willing to be consulted for future news stories, features, or opinion pieces.

Personal contact is even better, so don't hesitate to call a reporter. Remember, reporters make their living by talking to people. Tell the reporter who you are, what your background is, and what your specialties are. Be succinct; never waste a reporter's time. Once you've introduced yourself and your areas of interest, ask to arrange a future meeting. Some reporters like to make lunch or breakfast dates to meet with new sources; others prefer to keep meetings shorter and less formal.

When you meet the reporter, take advantage of the opportunity to discuss upcoming events, future story ideas, or reactions you and your colleagues have had to stories written by that reporter in the past. (The best way to flatter reporters is to let them know that you have read what they have written!) Again, let them know your areas of expertise and tell them you will be able to provide information in those areas in the future.

Some guidelines to keep in mind when you are talking to a journalist working on a story.

- Help answer the question the journalist is pursuing, even if you're not comfortable with his or her framing of the story, but then suggest another angle for the story. Even if you fail to redirect it, help with the story. The reporter will be back, and you'll get another chance.

239

- Keep in mind how you would like to see the article framed. Articulate and return to the three or four key points you want to stress.
- Have in mind a key bite (*see* Interview strategies): the one phrase you would like to see in print, either as a quote, or, even better, in the journalist's own words or as a headline.
- Rather than stretch your expertise, help reporters find the right expert. Be prepared to suggest other sources to help journalists prepare their stories: effective spokespeople who will help frame the issue well. A dilemma here can be what to do if the journalist asks your advice on who to interview for the "other side". Should you offer the names of those in your opposition whom you regard as being their most capable spokespeople? Or should you refer the journalist to your opposition's most inept representatives? One view is that you should avoid the temptation to steer reporters to ineffective opposition spokespeople whose poor performances will make your side look stronger. Those who hold to this view argue that when journalists realise that you may have set them up with a weaker "other" side to the story they are preparing, they will not thank you for having manipulated them and may well not come back to you on later occasions. If you sense (as often occurs) that the journalist is sympathetic to your cause, they may be only too willing to allow your opposition to portray their case in a deleterious way.
- Be willing *not* to be quoted—for example, if you are critical of lack of community consultation in a community health initiative, and you are a professional who doesn't live in the community in question, suggest a local community representative be interviewed. If you direct the journalist to good sources, journalists will remember this and come back to you next time.

Journalists and editors can have short memories. Although you will probably have a special interest in the media coverage that has been given to your public health issue over recent years, it is likely that you will encounter many journalists who have only a superficial acquaintance with your issue. Although you may live and breathe the memory of particular legislative battles, legal cases, or lobbying campaigns, a journalist may never have heard of such incidents. Many journalists in my experience are quite young (early 20s) and so would still have been at school or even not born when you may have been at the frontline on some aspect of your issue.

This observation applies also to research findings. In the early 1980s I issued a press release that challenged the tobacco industry to name the chemical additives that were being used to flavour, preserve, and regulate the burning temperature of cigarettes. The subtexts of the issue were "cover up and secretiveness by industry" and the related issue of the public's right to product information. The release attracted significant media coverage. In subsequent years, I have resurrected the same issue at least twice in deliberate releases and on several other occasions in response to slow news day "fishing expeditions" (when journalists phone regular news sources to see if they have any potential news stories simmering).

On each of these subsequent occasions, I have used virtually the same source material, the same framing of the issues involved, and the same sound bites. No journalist has ever said to me, "That's an old story", but have run the stories as if they were quite original. If you are contemplating resurrecting old stories, be advised that major newspapers will have files on each issue that could well be searched by the journalist for background material. If you are being overly repetitive or have not been straightforward with the journalist about the story being an old one, you may risk losing your credibility. None the less, all public health advocates have similar tales to tell about stories that seem to be irresistible to the press.

Create your own press list. Even if it only contains a handful of entries at the beginning, each should include the following information: name; title; publication; issue areas covered; address; phone and fax numbers; and any idiosyncrasies that may be relevant to your issue (for example, the reporter may have had a relative killed by a drunk driver; have mentioned that they have a relative affected by a disease you are working to prevent or care for; may have a reputation for liking to attend press meetings where there is plenty of food and drink; and so on).

As news stories develop, make use of your press list and maintain your press relationships by contacting them with new information, story ideas, and good leads. If you have close contacts with one or a few key journalists, you may want to offer them "exclusive" stories.

Finally, keep a copy of every story you help to generate. This will also help to determine whom you should contact for follow up and related future stories. In addition, sharing your successes with others can make it easier for them to generate publicity in their own communities. After all, once a story is reported, it is old news only to the paper that reported it. To all other media outlets, it may still be an opportunity.

Shareholders

If your opposition is a commercial company listed on the stock exchange, take the trouble to make lists of the directors and major shareholders of the company. These can serve as useful references for your understanding of the web of vested interests that are likely to support your opposition. Make special note of any significant joint directorships—for example, newspapers, broadcasting, and hospital boards—which might raise the public's eyebrows over suggestions of social control or hypocrisy. Such facts can speak for themselves when raised in a wry "well, what a coincidence!" fashion.

Public declarations by reputable groups that they will not invest in a particular company or industry for ethical reasons can be newsworthy and may cause other groups to reflect on their position. Shareholders may try to justify their stake by feebly arguing that it is of "a pure investment nature" and that they are not suggesting that they approve of the company or its product. This apathy speaks for itself.

Some public health advocates buy a small number of shares in their opposition's companies. The chief advantages of this are that it will place you on their mailing list for annual reports, new share listings, and news of the company. It will also allow you to attend shareholder meetings and functions such as annual general meetings. Such attendances can be used to great advocacy advantage if embarrassing questions are asked from the floor. Reporters often attend these meetings and your presence may provide good copy.[44] If different members of your coalition each buy shares and attend the shareholders meetings, your

Case study: shareholders

In 1985, David Player, then Director General of the British Health Education Council, funded the public interest group, Social Audit, to compile a list of tobacco shareholders in Britain whose investment in tobacco was ethically questionable. Player believed that if news got out to the public that groups concerned with health were having a bet on tobacco both ways, that many of the public would see this as hypocritical and the overall effort against tobacco would suffer. Shareholdings of public companies can be searched by computer. Key words such as "doctor", "royal", "medical", "hospital", "children" were submitted to the computer and a massive list emerged. These were listed in a special report published by the British Medical Association[43] under the following headings:

- Institutions in health and related areas
- Organisations concerned with children's welfare
- Educational establishments
- Church and related organisations
- Agencies involved in welfare and relief work
- Official and national agencies
- Local government authorities
- Pension funds.

Initially, a suggestion was made to write to all the shareholders listed in the report before its publication, suggesting that they may wish to review their policy in light of the health effects of tobacco. But in the heat of the revelations, this suggestion was not taken up and the report was published and covered widely by the press. Predictably, this led to a mixed reaction. Some groups named declared publicly that they would be selling all their tobacco shares whereas others were drawn into justifying their retention. But the worst result was undoubtedly the public scrap that ensued between a cancer charity with shares and the BMA, the former accusing the latter of not consulting them and implying a motive of humiliation. Anyone contemplating a similar exercise should definitely keep their findings private until shareholding groups have at least been given a chance to reconsider. Otherwise it is likely to be a case of "divide and rule" in your opposition's favour.

protest questions will not appear to be coming only from individuals but from a seemingly larger number of shareholders seated throughout the meeting.

Slow news days

In an important way, news should be understood as a product manufactured by the news gathering process. This means that at times when there are fewer people actually gathering news, there will be correspondingly fewer news stories being gathered and competing for the limited space in print, radio, or television news outlets. At such times, the chances of any given story being both picked up by a reporter and published are much higher than normal. The chances are made even greater by the correspondence of slow news gathering periods with lower activity periods in the community generally. Weekends, particularly Sundays, public holidays, and summer holiday periods are the most obvious slow news days that can be exploited. Remember also that these times can be disastrous times to stage press conferences: skeleton staff operate in many media and, if a bigger story than yours breaks, these staff will probably be drawn away from yours and it is unlikely that substitute journalists will be available to take over. At the end of the day there is no foolproof way of guaranteeing that a bigger story than yours will not break: it's just that the probability of this not happening is bigger on slow news days.

Strategic research

It is important to anticipate how research might enhance your advocacy objectives. Is your opposition constantly alluding to community support for their position? Do you suspect that this support is not all it seems? Is there a critical piece of missing information or perspective that, were it available, might dramatically alter the terms in which an issue is being debated? Most areas of public health advocacy have several such gaps and the strategic use of research to plug them is a very common tactic used by advocates.

244

The results from small surveys, often conducted in convenience samples, can often be picked up by the media as "snapshot" hooks on which to hang a story. Journalists and editors are not statisticians, survey specialists, or epidemiologists, and consequently will tend not to assess data from a "survey" in the way you may be used to when writing for scientific journals. Standard errors, confidence intervals, and significance tests may preoccupy your colleagues, but they will seldom if ever make any difference to the way the media reports the results of a survey or poll. The advantages of this to public health advocacy can just as easily be seen as advantages to your opposition and there are many examples of the enemies of public health torpedoing policy initiatives by issuing the results of quick and dirty research of very questionable validity.

It should be emphasised that the risks of losing credibility both within your own professional or community constituency and with the media by conducting or promoting shoddy research are great indeed. Strategic research should *never* be understood as a synonym for poor quality research. Nearly every piece of research, however, has the potential to snake down a myriad of inconsequential and confusing pathways determined by over-cautiousness or an overly zealous respect for comprehensiveness. Strategic research can often be simple, conducted quickly and of high quality within the objectives set for it.

Case study: strategic research

Philip Morris in Australia argued persistently that its small, inexpensive packs of 15 cigarettes were not marketed with children in mind, despite an overtly teenage oriented advertising campaign. A quick survey comparing schoolchildren and adults from the same area showed otherwise: 57% of smoking children had bought a pack of 15s in the past month compared with only 8% of adult smokers.[45] As a result, Philip Morris's argument was quickly diffused and the small packs banned in South Australia,[46] causing a domino effect around all the other Australian states in the following few years.

245

Case study: strategic research

In the lead up to the 1993 Australian Federal elections, the Government argued strongly that the conservative Opposition's deregulated health policy would result in doctors raising their fees, causing hardship and underuse of medical services by the poor. The Opposition denied that this would happen, and the Australian Medical Association (which openly supported the Opposition) similarly issued strong denials from their national office.

The Doctors' Reform Society, a small group of doctors committed to the retention of the Government's "bulk-billing" policy (whereby doctors bill the Government instead of patients for medical services), conducted a survey of all 42 general practitioners working in a marginal electoral seat held narrowly by the Opposition's shadow health minister (see Marginal seats). Seventy eight per cent of the 42 doctors claimed that they would raise their fees if the Opposition were elected. The survey results were reported as the page one lead story in the *Sydney Morning Herald* three days before the election.[47] The story was headlined "DOCTORS SAY THEY'LL RAISE FEES IF HEWSON [the Opposition leader] WINS", thus framing the small survey as if it could somehow be taken to be representative of doctors at large. The story dominated news debate about the election all that day and was so big that it went onto the front page the next day too, with a profile of one doctor who confirmed the likely rise in fees.[48] The Doctor's Reform Society had conducted a legitimate piece of strategic research in one urban area and had calculated (correctly) that the press would be less concerned with questions of its generalisability than with its potential as a concrete snapshot of doctors' views.

Talent (spokespeople)

In Chapters 2 and 3, we looked at the types of people favoured by journalists as news sources. The media refer to news actors (those who make news) as "talent", a reference that reflects the essentially dramaturgic nature of the way media workers conceive of news. Many public health causes feature spokespeople who are so distractingly bad in some aspect of their presentation that they all but destroy any advantage their issue may have in media representations. Broadcast journalists who judge you as poor talent will be very reluctant ever to call on you again. The result can be an avoidable neglect of your issue, simply because of its identification with you as someone who is difficult to work with or who will bore audiences and the journalists themselves. On the other hand, an engaging, articulate, credible, and skilled media advocate can attract inordinate positive attention to an issue, way beyond that which someone regarded as having less "talent" might.

Many organisations assume that the importance of a media appearance warrants the most senior person in the organisation being the obvious spokesperson to deal with the media. The Advocacy Institute comments:

Your best spokesperson may or may not be you—or the boss. The head of your organisation may be the right name on a press release, or the named author of an op-ed [opinion] article, but not an experienced or effective broadcast presence. Your organisational culture may encourage volunteers to speak for the organisation while professional staff members are expected to remain in the background. That may be a fine practice for many occasions—but not for handling a professionally trained adversary. Of course, choosing the right spokesperson sometimes requires exquisite tact and considerable courage.[2]

If your issue or organisation is one that is labouring under the burden of an inappropriate spokesperson, especially one who is in a managerial or executive role, it may be possible to address this issue through the services of an outside media consultant, whose independence may allow them to make the point that underlings within the organisation cannot. Equally, instituting some form of evaluation of media performances through focus groups of either members of the public or relevant experts may produce information and feedback that will be useful. Finally, the acid test of how well your organisation's "talent" is viewed by the media will be the extent to which the media return for comment on other occasions, especially in relation to news stories where they have some discretion on whom to interview.

The smoking control lobby occasionally labours under the unfortunate public image legacy of some of its early activists, many of whom were the last word in puritanism and everything that represents dullness. To such people, smoking was a self-indulgent evil and tobacco the devil's weed. Smoking was a symptom of some more fundamental moral turpitude and so it was smokers, more than smoking, that was at the heart of what they reviled. Think about the characteristic vaudeville representation of the non-smoker and imagine most people's response to a word association exercise using "anti-smoker" and it's easy to see some of the difficulties that still beset the field today. Many probably still believe that, given some rein, people taking a stance against smoking would like to stop everyone drinking, lace everyone up, turn the music down at your party, take all sweets out of children's mouths, and ban sex, and probably laughing, too. How many who might otherwise stop and think about smoking dismiss or relegate the message because of this pious and totally unnecessary wrapper?

Talkback (access) radio

Talkback radio (when radio broadcasters open their programme to listeners who phone in and talk on air) can provide a host of opportunities for you to place a message in front of mass audiences at no cost. The talkback genre is meant to create the illusion of a form of random sampling of public views on issues. It is radio's equivalent of the way newspapers sometimes run a series of *vox pop* one-line responses to a news item by people intercepted in shopping malls. Talkback is seen by radio programmers as something different to the soliciting of expert or lobby group views on an issue. Talkback occasionally features people with authority or expertise phoning in, but generally, it is seen by stations as an access medium for the person in the street. This means that you should probably treat it in the way it is intended to function and identify yourself as simply a person with a view on the issue being discussed. Alternatively, you can describe yourself as someone with some special interest or expertise in the issue—for example, "Hello, I'm a doctor, and I've been listening to some of your callers arguing that food labelling is confusing. I'd like to tell you about a patient of mine with an allergy to . . ." It is best to avoid being seen as a member of a lobby group trying to exploit the medium. The station's attitude is likely to be one of wanting to control such groups' access through an invitation to be interviewed.

Although many callers to talkback radio are genuine, unaffiliated, "ordinary" people, a surprising number would probably turn out to be rather more calculating. Many political parties and lobby groups deliberately try to "stack" talkback programmes in attempts to convey to listeners that there is widespread support for their issue or position. It is common practice, for example, for staffers in politicians' offices to use up any spare moments trying to phone through calls to talkback programmes. This occurs especially when the politician they work for is in the studio taking calls (here, they feed preferred questions and ladle out praise) or when the political opposition is there (here, they go on the attack).

The important thing to remember is that neither the radio host nor the audience has any way of knowing that a caller is anything more than just that: an ordinary person with an opinion. If these opinions can be articulated with reference to the key principles discussed throughout this book, and if they appear to be coming in from the public one after the other, valuable advocacy reaching thousands or sometimes millions of people can occur.

Getting on air

As anyone who has tried to get through to a talkback programme knows, it is often difficult—all lines are usually full. Knowing this, many callers telephone the programme in advance and have been waiting on the line, unbeknown to listeners, for up to 20 minutes. You must be prepared to do this too. This means that you must know when the talkback segment of different radio programmes usually starts or when the host announces what the subject of that day's talkback will be (some stations have "open line" talkback, where any subject can be raised by listeners). Assuming the former, you can then decide whether on that day it will be worth your while telephoning through. If there is a big news story breaking around your issue, the chances that it will be covered on talkback are greater than normal. It may be wise to activate the first few limbs of your telephone tree if a talkback session looks promising (*see* Telephone trees).

When you telephone through, your call will be answered by a programme researcher or producer. Generally, this person will ask you your first name and what it is that you want to talk about. Keywords from this information will often be keyed into a monitor visible to the radio host in the studio. Sometimes, the host will not go to air with the calls in the order they come in, but rather choose calls that balance one another. Others use the monitor to screen out callers with views they don't want to broadcast. If this is working against your issue, you can only know about this from experience. If it happens, you may decide that the only way to get on air is to appear to have changed your mind about what you want to say when you are actually talking to the host on air.

It is a good idea to draw up a week's calendar of all radio stations, marking each day with the stations that run talkback programmes during particular hours. Code or somehow note against each programme anything that might be important to your issue—for example, host known to be sympathetic or antagonistic to your cause. To save time looking up station telephone numbers and fumbling with the dial, pre-set radio station access lines into your office telephones to ensure that your call can get through.

Targeting or narrowcasting

Sending a message through the airwaves to reach as many people as possible is called "broadcasting"; targeting the audiences that you need to reach through the right medium is called "narrowcasting". When you are seeking to persuade active citizens or community leaders to support your policies, it is important to target your media initiatives to those media that your target audience reads or views, and respects, and to frame and express your position in ways that will elicit the best response from the target group with whom you are most concerned. Effective media advocacy starts with an understanding of how an issue relates to the prevailing public opinions and values of your target group; only then can media messages be designed that will broaden an advocate's base of public support.

Research can help advocates determine how the public views various issues and symbols. Even fairly simple, low cost research can help monitor public attitudes and perceptions within your community. National polls can also help reveal which of your policy initiatives is misconceived or distorted by segments of the public, and therefore needs symbolic reframing. Qualitative research, such as focus groups, is another useful tool for indicating how the public feels about issues and symbols. Armed with an understanding of the public's dominant concerns, advocates can successfully begin to frame an issue.

When developing your messages, keep your target audience firmly in mind. Constantly ask yourself if the message being formulated is likely to be appropriate for the chosen group. An anti-tobacco message designed for policy makers will probably not be effective for reaching adolescents.

In using any particular media outlet, you need to understand what kind of language and tone that audience responds to. The audience for a local public radio channel may be far more interested in scientific discourse than those who enjoy the combative give and take of a local call-in talk show. As a result, it is your responsibility to make sure that your media advocacy message is suited for your audience.

For example, if you were presenting a speech to convince a Mothers Against Drunk Driving (MADD) group to support a local initiative, your message would be markedly different than the same speech presented in front of a group of civic leaders with no established position on alcohol control.

Just as your message must be tailored to the specific audience you have in mind, you must also adjust your material to the medium that you use. A commercial that sells through visual appeal on television is not going to be effective on the radio. Similarly, a wordy magazine advertisement would not be as effective on a billboard. In short, each medium has varying strengths and weaknesses which you should keep in mind as you formulate your media advocacy strategy (for more detail on this, see Chapter 2).

251

Case study: framing in targeting

The pro-choice (concerning abortion) movement has long recognised the need to use symbols that resonate with the public. They continually seek ways to make their message more appealing to a broader spectrum of the population. Says Judith Lichtman, of the Women's Legal Defense Fund, "We have changed our rhetoric from talking about body integrity, which didn't work, to talking about choice, which does." Although body integrity seemed a perfect message to Washington activists, their research determined that it did not sell "outside" Washington. In order to get their message across to the electorate as a whole (not just to their supporters), they had to frame it differently. By focusing on a woman's right to choose, they have positioned themselves in the mainstream, while portraying their opponents as out of the mainstream.

Even with this useful message, the pro-choice movement has sought more ways to tailor the pro-choice message to the public's concerns:

- Pro-choice advocates learned through focus groups that their paid advertisements (predicting that if abortion were made illegal, women and doctors could go to jail) just did not convince people. The public realised that with full jails and courts, it was highly unlikely that women who underwent an abortion would be jailed. On the other hand, the advocates found a message that did work: people feared that making abortions illegal would mean that they would be performed in illegal settings, and that was a convincing argument for keeping abortions legal. The groups would never have discovered this point of view without the use of focus groups.

- Despite a heavy investment in polling and focus groups, a Michigan pro-choice coalition failed to heed the direction indicated by that information. The pro-choice group's public opinion information revealed that the public was antagonistic to those on welfare, believing that they abused the system. Contrary to what the pro-choice advocates thought among themselves, the public was unmoved by the plight of poor women who had been raped or been the victims of incest. Yet in their media advertisements, the advocates still raised the plight of poor women. Partly for this reason, their pro-choice advocacy failed.

Editorial pages are usually far less well read than "style" sections of local newspapers but they are read intensely by the community leaders who help shape public policy. In many countries, public broadcasting stations have smaller audiences than commercial stations but reach large segments of those active citizens whom political scientists call the "attentive public."

By using the appropriate medium, you can reach your targeted audience. For example, if you want to reach people in the medical profession, there are a variety of periodicals that cater to medical professionals only, and a number that target members of specific medical specialties. Spreading your message in these periodicals would help you to reach your specific audience and therefore to accomplish your media advocacy goals.

At times, it is appropriate to use widely read and widely viewed media judiciously to reach a narrow audience. Consider the 1987 campaign to stop the right wing Robert Bork's nomination to the US Supreme Court.[41] The anti-Bork coalition knew that its ultimate audience was the Senate Judiciary Committee, which had the responsibility for deciding whether Reagan's nominee was appropriate for the nation's highest court. To reach the senators on that committee, and especially the handful of "swing" votes, the coalition knew it must use media that would reach those senators as well as media that would reach their constituents. On a few broadcast news shows sure to be seen by those senators and on the local news of key constituents, the coalition ran a 60 second television spot featuring Gregory Peck talking about Bork's dismal civil rights record. Peck warns: "Robert Bork could have the last word on your rights as a citizen. But, the Senate has the last word on him. Please urge your Senators to vote against the Bork nomination . . ."

As media advocate Dr Anne Marie O'Keefe points out, this message sounds like it is aimed at all viewers, but in fact it was directly aimed at a few key senators and their constituents. Rather than spending millions of dollars on a national media blitz, the coalition ran the spot just 20 times, keeping its advertising costs to a minimum. The Gregory Peck spot cost just $160 000. As the anti-Bork campaign demonstrated, narrowcasting can help a campaign win efficiently.

It is important to be aware of who you believe to be your most important media audience. As you develop your media advocacy

253

projects, identify your target audience. Ask yourself at whom your media advocacy strategy should be targeted. Do you want to reach the general public? How about policy makers? Do you only want your message to be tailored to activists already on your side? Or do you want to target people who are "on the fence" and could be easily persuaded to take action for your cause?

Telephone trees

Telephone trees are arrangements whereby advocates use the principle of geometric progression to alert supporters to a proposed course of action. They work in the way chain letters do. The following illustration shows how they can work. A politician informs your office that he or she would like to receive urgently an avalanche of letters of support for a legislative proposal. You immediately telephone or fax five of your members, asking them to write a short letter of support and, in turn, each to telephone five of their friends or colleagues, asking them to do the same, and so on. By the time this process reaches only its fourth generation, a cumulative total of 781 letters could be on their way within a couple of hours of you having received the call from the politician. Naturally, this process will not yield 100% compliance from everyone called, but even with a fractional success, a formidable number of people can be drawn into taking action.

Telephone trees will work best if you ensure that:

- The first people you call are strong supporters of your cause and known to be reliable in their willingness to make the quota of calls that are necessary.
- Those on the lower branches of the tree are similarly known to be reliable in passing on their quota of calls.
- You aim to select people on these lower branches who are as diverse as possible—for example, health workers, academics, community groups, industry and commerce people, and church leaders. If your lower branches are all from similar backgrounds, it is more likely that the callers up the tree will soon start turning back on people who have already been called by others.

Telephone trees can be used to get people to demonstrations at short notice, to make telephone calls or write letters, to attend emergency meetings, and so on.

Whistleblowers

Whistleblowers (people who break ranks from their expected duty of confidentiality and give the "inside story"—usually about corruption, duplicity, or dirty dealings) hold immense fascination for the media. Whistleblowers carry with them subtexts of bravery, uncommonness, and telling the truth, which gives them intrinsic newsworthiness. Whistleblowers can be anyone from very senior people in organisations right down to humble workers who have witnessed "things going on" that they feel the public should know about. Disgruntled or disaffected relatives or partners of people in organisations also sometimes blow the whistle.

Rather than waiting for whistleblowers to take the initiative, it can be an interesting exercise to advertise that you are interested in having confidential discussions with people who may be sympathetic with your objectives (*see* Infiltration).

Wolves in sheep's clothing

If your opposition has been having a credibility crisis with the media, it may have resorted to the common strategy of funding and supporting seemingly "independent" community and business groups who will do its bidding, untainted by having any direct connection with them.[34] These groups typically have names that incorporate sound, respectable values, the idea being to render attacks on their particular positions as attacks on the invincible values behind which they seek to shelter. The tobacco industry has an impressive record of funding and otherwise supporting such groups, particularly around the passive smoking issue. Some of these groups include the Freedom Organisation for the Right to Enjoy Smoking Tobacco (FOREST), Citizens Against More Tax and Bureaucracy,[35] the California Business and Restaurant Alliance, Californians for Fair Business Policy, Restaurants for a Sensible Voluntary Policy, and Healthy

Case study: whistleblowers

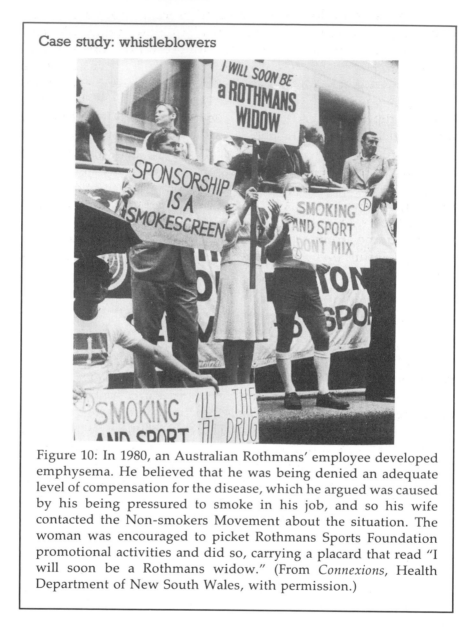

Figure 10: In 1980, an Australian Rothmans' employee developed emphysema. He believed that he was being denied an adequate level of compensation for the disease, which he argued was caused by his being pressured to smoke in his job, and so his wife contacted the Non-smokers Movement about the situation. The woman was encouraged to picket Rothmans Sports Foundation promotional activities and did so, carrying a placard that read "I will soon be a Rothmans widow." (From *Connexions*, Health Department of New South Wales, with permission.)

Buildings International, the latter a regular front for the industry and subject of a searing piece of investigative journalism in *The Nation*.[49]

As discussed under Talent, the credibility of those seen to be delivering a message can be critical to how believable and persuasive they are seen to be. Your opposition will often seek to frame or label you in some pejorative way. The objective here is to distract audiences from considering what you are saying, by making them become preoccupied by who you are or the values that you represent. Front groups, cloaked in the respectability of a label such as "freedom" or "fairness" can step into a debate with you with a head start in the eyes of an unsuspecting audience.

If you suspect that a group is being funded by your opposition, investigate the connection and, if it is confirmed, use this information ruthlessly. If you are successful, you may quickly shift the frame around their respectable presence to the probably more powerful one of deception and the "wolf in sheep's clothing."

Wrestling with pigs

The idea that there is a "debate" about particular public health issues is a notion that many opponents of public health are very glad to perpetuate. A debate implies that the jury is still out, that there are "two sides", when often the public health implications of the issue at stake are patently obvious. There are some who argue that to join in public media debates with such people is to legitimise their arguments and that it is preferable not to rise to the bait, taking your media opportunities at your own deciding. When your opposition goes public, however, an absence of response by health and consumer representatives may be taken as a sign of you not having an answer, of defeat.

Dr Alan Blum of Doctors Ought to Care (DOC) in Houston, Texas, is one who argues that debates with opposition groups should be generally avoided. Blum argues, "When you wrestle with pigs, you both get dirty—but the pig loves it!" He argues that, if your opposition mouthpiece succeeds in dragging down the level of public discourse to a shouting match between two equally unappealing zealots, and you are one of them, your cause will suffer. With your public health aims and objectives firmly in view, give consideration to whether the probability of such an

257

encounter will be in the best interests of these objectives. Balance any decision to withdraw from, or decline, a debate with your opposition against the likelihood of the subtext framing your absence that says to the public you were "too afraid/had something to hide/were avoiding confrontation with hard facts", and so on.

If you do go ahead and debate, point out during the debate that your opponent is a paid agent whose job is to protect his industry's profits or her government employer's policy. Suggest that he or she will be in trouble if they don't toe the expected line. Refer to what they say in terms such as "the company song", "beginning to sound like a cracked record", and so on. Cajole them, as human beings, to drop the act and speak "off the record". Of course they will not, but your raising the idea that the opposition person is just parroting a line and is insincere will cause many to reassess what they are saying.

Xmas

Christmas is one of the slowest of slow news periods in the year (*see* Slow news days) and can be a good time to gain access to the media. Over Christmas, people are at leisure and an article in the media can attract a larger than normal audience or readership as people take more time to read a newspaper or laze in front of television. Christmas carries with it particular associations that can provide useful hooks to a range of public health advocacy issues. As a time of family togetherness, giving, receiving, and sharing, it can serve as a poignant reminder of those for whom Christmas is a time of isolation and loneliness, or a time when thoughtless excess could otherwise be channelled into donating money to a socially worthwhile cause.

References

1 Chapman S. *The lung goodbye. Tactics for counteracting the tobacco industry in the 1980s.* Consumer Interpol: Sydney, 1986, 2nd ed.
2 Pertschuk M, Wilbur P. *Media advocacy: strategies for reframing public debate.* Washington DC: The Advocacy Institute, 1990.

3 The Advocacy Institute. *Getting through to the front page.* Washington DC: The Advocacy Institute, 1990.

4 Baum FE. Healthy cities and change: social movement or bureaucratic tool? *Health Promotion Int* 1993; **8**: 31–40.

5 Wilkes MS, Kravitz RL. Medical researchers and the media. Attitudes toward public dissemination of research. *JAMA* 1992; **268**: 999–1003.

6 Chapman S. Competing agenda in smoking control agencies . . . Those who pay the piper. *NY State J Med* 1985; **85**: 287–9.

7 Sethi SP. *Advocacy advertising and large corporations.* Lexington, MA: Lexington Books, 1977.

8 Pertschuk M. Smoking gun speaks: the tobacco industry's Buy America strategy. *ANR Update* 1992; **12**(3): 3.

9 Alinsky S. *Rules for radicals.* New York: Vintage, 1972.

10 Allain A. *IBFAN on the cutting edge.* Oslo: Dag Hammarskjold Foundation, 1991.

11 Statistical Consulting Unit, School of Mathematics, Queensland University of Technology. *Factors affecting fatal road crash trends. Report for Federal Office of Road Safety, Canberra, ACT, Australia.* June 1992.

12 Lagan B. Fuel price cut will lift road toll, says study. *Sydney Morning Herald* 1993 March 6; 9.

13 Gribben R. BAT man who answered the call for help. *Daily Telegraph* 1993 July 1; 4.

14 Masters R. The damning graph that killed tobacco sponsorship. *Sydney Morning Herald* 1992 April 2; 1.

15 Vollmer T. How far the politics of anger? *San Francisco Sentinel* 1990 June 28; 9.

16 Vollmer T. Three points for ACT UP to consider. *San Francisco Sentinel* 1990 Aug 2; 9.

17 Hagon W. Car race teams give up smokes. *Sunday Telegraph* 1985 24 Feb.

18 Cover. *Med J Aust.* 1982: July 24.

19 Fitzsimons P. Health body slams League poll claim. *Sydney Morning Herald* 1991 Nov 13; 62.

20 Wachter RM. *The fragile coalition: scientists, activists, and AIDS.* New York: St Martin's Press, 1991.

21 Hippocratic corpus, decorum. In: Reiser SJ, Dyck AF, Curran WJ (editors). *Ethics in medicine: historical perspectives and contemporary concerns.* Cambridge, MA: MIT Press, 1977: 7.

22 Osler W. Aequanimitas with other addresses: internal medicine as a vocation. Philadelphia, PA: P Blakiston & Son, 1905.

23 DeVries WC. The physician, the media, and the 'spectacular' case. *JAMA* 1988; **259**: 886–90.

24 Angell M, Kassirer JP. The Ingelfinger rule revisited. *N Engl J Med* 1991; **323**: 1371–3.

25 Relman AS. The Ingelfinger rule. *N Engl J Med* 1981; **305**: 824–6.

26 Brass A. Smoke gets in your eyes. *Med J Aust* 1984; **140**: 459.

27 Ragg M. To win, start stroking the media. *Medical Observer* 1992 Oct 1.

28 McCann D. Dentistry in the headlines: the profession and the press. *J Am Dent Assoc* 1990; **120**: 483–90.

29 Bloom J. Fear and irony on tobacco road: notes from the Fourth Tobacco International Exhibition and Conference. *Tobacco Control* 1993; **2**: 46–9.

30 Di Franza JR, Brown LJ. The Tobacco Institute's 'It's the law' campaign: has it halted illegal sales of tobacco to children? *Am J Public Health* 1992; **82**: 1271–3.

31 Walsh G. Postscript. *Sydney Morning Herald* 1993 Aug 30; 14.

32 Garcia LM. School anti-smoking material attacked as 'propaganda'. *Sydney Morning Herald* 1985 Apr 30.

33 Wood AA. The aims of cigarette advertising (letter). *Sydney Morning Herald* 1983 Aug 25.

34 Samuels B, Glantz SA. The politics of local tobacco control. *JAMA* 1991; **266**: 2110–17.

35 Moon RW, Males MA, Nelson DE. The 1990 Montana initiative to increase cigarette taxes: lessons or other states and localities. *J Public Health Policy* 1993; **14**: 19–32.

36 Marr M. *Proposition 99: the California Tobacco Tax Initiative, a Case Study.* Berkeley, CA: Western Consortium for Public Health, 1990.

37 Advocacy Institute. *Taking initiative: the 1990 citizen's movement to raise California alcohol excise taxes to save lives.* Washington: The Advocacy Institute, 1992.

38 Chapman S. Anatomy of a campaign: the attempt to defeat the NSW Tobacco Advertising Prohibition Bill 1991. *Tobacco Control* 1992; **1**: 50–6.

39 Taylor L, Eccleston R. Anti-gun lobby wants ad axed. *The Australian* 1993 Feb 13–14; 1, 12.

40 Australian Council on Smoking and Health. *Tobacco Company Alternative Report* 1987. Perth: ACOSH, 1987.

41 Pertschuk M, Schaetzel W. *The people rising. The campaign against the Bork nomination.* New York: Thunder's Mouth Press, 1989.

42 Wachter RM. AIDS, activism, and the politics of health. *N Engl J Med* 1992; **326**: 128–33.

43 Gilbert D. *Report on investment in the UK tobacco industry.* London: British Medical Association Professional Division, Jan 1985.

44 Blum A. Cowboys, cancer, kids, and cash flow: the 1992 Philip Morris annual meeting. *Tobacco Control* 1992; **1**: 134–7.

45 Wilson DH, Wakefield MA, Esterman A, Baker CC. 15s: They fit in everywhere, especially the schoolbag. *Community Health Stud* 1987; suppl. 11(1): 16–20.

46 Chapman S, Reynolds C. Regulating tobacco—The South Australian Tobacco Products Control Act 1986. *Community Health Stud* 1987; suppl. 11(1): 9–15.

47 Larriera A. Doctors say they'll raise fees if Hewson wins. *Sydney Morning Herald* 1993 March 10; 1.

48 Larriera A, Date M. Doctor warns of fee dilemma under Liberals. *Sydney Morning Herald* 1993 March 11; 1.

49 Levin M. Who's behind the building door? *The Nation* 1993 Aug 9–16; 168–71.

Index

menstruation 68
mental health 29
Mercedes Benz company 227
messages 49-53, 251
  unplanned 24
metaphors 141
Mitchell, Warren 148
MOP UP 138, 164-5, 166
moral tales 64-7
Ms 31

narrowcasting 250-4
National Health and Medical
    Research Council 201
National Portrait Gallery 168
Nelson, Brendon 143
networks 219-20
  computer 220
New Delhi 183
*New England Journal of
    Medicine* 33, 36, 136, 172,
    234
New Idea 76, 80
news
  actors 45-7, 246-7
  doctors 65-6
  production 29-30
  selection 32
  social construction 29-31
  sources 45-7
  story structure 44
  values 28-9
news bulletin (Channel 7,
    Sydney) 193, 194
news coverage 23
  audience response 49-53
  content analysis 37-8
  discourse analysis 38-49
  journalists' perspective 33-7
  power of advertisers 30-1
  unplanned messsages 24
newsgathering 19, 244
news media 27-8
  cultures 19
  messages 19-20

power 24-7
role 17-18
pluralistic value 69
News of the World 84
newspapers 28, 34-5, 50, 92-3
  British stories 82-91
  censorship 13
  columnists 158
  editorials 174-5
  letters 199-204, 220, 221
  local 208-9
  opinion pages 222-3
  Sydney stories 70-3, 74-82
Newsweek 28, 49, 73
newsworthiness 18
  principles 31-3
Newton-John, Olivia 153
New York State 24
New York Times 33, 35, 226
Nile, Fred 114
non-governmental
    organisations 137, 152

obesity clinic 68
Observer 89
O'Keefe, Anne Marie 253
opinion pages 222-3
opinion polls 223-4
opinions 45 7
opportunism 224-7
opposition
  binary 93
  debate with 257-8
  funding groups 255-7
  infiltration 181-3
  knowing 197
  mailing lists 209-10
  quotes 234-5
  power 11-12
  response 208
oral health 29
Osler, William 172
Otten, Alan 18
overkill 105